Motor Neurone Disease

Dr David Oliver trained as a GP and worked at St Christopher's Hospice in London before becoming Consultant in Palliative Medicine and Medical Director at the Wisdom Hospice in Rochester. He is also Honorary Senior Lecturer at the Centre for Professional Practice in the University of Kent, and Visiting Professor at the Medical Faculty of the University of Zagreb in Croatia. He has been closely involved in the care of people with motor neurone disease (MND) and has spoken and written widely on their care and the management of symptoms. In 2003 he was awarded the Humanitarian Award by the International Alliance of Amyotrophic Lateral Sclerosis (ALS)/MND Associations in recognition of his role in education across the world.

D1396422

Overcoming Common Problems Series

Selected titles

A full list of titles is available from Sheldon Press,
36 Causton Street, London SW1P 4ST and on our website at
www.sheldonpress.co.uk

Asperger Syndrome in Adults
Dr Ruth Searle

The Assertiveness Handbook
Mary Hartley

Assertiveness: Step by step
Dr Windy Dryden and Daniel Constantinou

Backache: What you need to know
Dr David Delvin

Body Language: What you need to know
David Cohen

Bulimia, Binge-eating and their Treatment
Professor J. Hubert Lacey, Dr Bryony Bamford and
Amy Brown

The Cancer Survivor's Handbook
Dr Terry Priestman

The Chronic Pain Diet Book
Neville Shone

Cider Vinegar
Margaret Hills

Confidence Works
Gladeana McMahon

Coping Successfully with Pain
Neville Shone

Coping Successfully with Prostate Cancer
Dr Tom Smith

Coping Successfully with Psoriasis
Christine Craggs-Hinton

Coping Successfully with Ulcerative Colitis
Peter Cartwright

Coping Successfully with Varicose Veins
Christine Craggs-Hinton

Coping Successfully with Your Hiatus Hernia
Dr Tom Smith

Coping Successfully with Your Irritable Bowel
Rosemary Nicol

Coping When Your Child Has Cerebral Palsy
Jill Eckersley

Coping with Age-related Memory Loss
Dr Tom Smith

**Coping with Birth Trauma and Postnatal
Depression**
Lucy Jolin

Coping with Bowel Cancer
Dr Tom Smith

Coping with Candida
Shirley Trickett

Coping with Chemotherapy
Dr Terry Priestman

Coping with Chronic Fatigue
Trudie Chalder

Coping with Coeliac Disease
Karen Brody

Coping with Compulsive Eating
Dr Ruth Searle

**Coping with Diabetes in Childhood and
Adolescence**
Dr Philippa Kaye

Coping with Diverticulitis
Peter Cartwright

Coping with Dyspraxia
Jill Eckersley

Coping with Early-onset Dementia
Jill Eckersley

Coping with Eating Disorders and Body Image
Christine Craggs-Hinton

Coping with Envy
Dr Windy Dryden

**Coping with Epilepsy in Children and Young
People**
Susan Elliot-Wright

Coping with Family Stress
Dr Peter Cheevers

Coping with Gout
Christine Craggs-Hinton

Coping with Hay Fever
Christine Craggs-Hinton

Coping with Headaches and Migraine
Alison Frith

Coping with Hearing Loss
Christine Craggs-Hinton

Coping with Heartburn and Reflux
Dr Tom Smith

Coping with Kidney Disease
Dr Tom Smith

Overcoming Common Problems Series

Coping with Life after Stroke
Dr Mareeni Raymond

Coping with Life's Challenges: Moving on from adversity
Dr Windy Dryden

Coping with Phobias and Panic
Professor Kevin Gournay

Coping with PMS
Dr Farah Ahmed and Dr Emma Cordle

Coping with Polycystic Ovary Syndrome
Christine Craggs-Hinton

Coping with Postnatal Depression
Sandra L. Wheatley

Coping with the Psychological Effects of Cancer
Professor Robert Bor, Dr Carina Eriksen and Ceilidh Stapelkamp

Coping with Radiotherapy
Dr Terry Priestman

Coping with Rheumatism and Arthritis
Dr Keith Souter

Coping with Snoring and Sleep Apnoea
Jill Eckersley

Coping with a Stressed Nervous System
Dr Kenneth Hambly and Alice Muir

Coping with Suicide
Maggie Helen

Coping with Tinnitus
Christine Craggs-Hinton

Coping with Type 2 Diabetes
Susan Elliot-Wright

Coping with Your Partner's Death: Your bereavement guide
Geoff Billings

Depression: Healing emotional distress
Linda Hurcombe

Depressive Illness
Dr Tim Cantopher

Divorce and Separation: A legal guide for all couples
Dr Mary Welstead

Dynamic Breathing: How to manage your asthma
Dinah Bradley and Tania Clifton-Smith

Every Woman's Guide to Digestive Health
Jill Eckersley

The Fertility Handbook
Dr Philippa Kaye

The Fibromyalgia Healing Diet
Christine Craggs-Hinton

Free Yourself from Depression
Colin and Margaret Sutherland

A Guide to Anger Management
Mary Hartley

Helping Children Cope with Anxiety
Jill Eckersley

Helping Children Cope with Grief
Rosemary Wells

High-risk Body Size: Take control of your weight
Dr Funké Baffour

How to Beat Pain
Christine Craggs-Hinton

How to Beat Worry and Stress
Dr David Delvin

How to Cope with Difficult People
Alan Houel and Christian Godefroy

How to Live with a Control Freak
Barbara Baker

How to Lower Your Blood Pressure: And keep it down
Christine Craggs-Hinton

How to Manage Chronic Fatigue
Christine Craggs-Hinton

Hysterectomy: Is it right for you?
Janet Wright

The IBS Healing Plan
Theresa Cheung

Living with Angina
Dr Tom Smith

Living with Asperger Syndrome
Dr Joan Gomez

Living with Autism
Fiona Marshall

Living with Bipolar Disorder
Dr Neel Burton

Living with Birthmarks and Blemishes
Gordon Lamont

Living with Crohn's Disease
Dr Joan Gomez

Living with Eczema
Jill Eckersley

Living with Fibromyalgia
Christine Craggs-Hinton

Living with Food Intolerance
Alex Gazzola

Living with Gluten Intolerance
Jane Feinmann

Living with Grief
Dr Tony Lake

Living with Loss and Grief
Julia Tugendhat

Overcoming Common Problems Series

Living with Osteoarthritis
Dr Patricia Gilbert

Living with Osteoporosis
Dr Joan Gomez

Living with Physical Disability and Amputation
Dr Keren Fisher

Living with a Problem Drinker: Your survival guide
Rolande Anderson

Living with Rheumatoid Arthritis
Philippa Pigache

Living with Schizophrenia
Dr Neel Burton and Dr Phil Davison

Living with a Seriously Ill Child
Dr Jan Aldridge

Living with Sjögren's Syndrome
Sue Dyson

Living with a Stoma
Professor Craig A. White

Living with Tinnitus and Hyperacusis
Dr Laurence McKenna, Dr David Baguley and Dr Don McFerran

Losing a Child
Linda Hurcombe

Menopause in Perspective
Philippa Pigache

The Multiple Sclerosis Diet Book
Tessa Buckley

Osteoporosis: Prevent and treat
Dr Tom Smith

Overcome Your Fear of Flying
Professor Robert Bor, Dr Carina Eriksen and Margaret Oakes

Overcoming Agoraphobia
Melissa Murphy

Overcoming Anorexia
Professor J. Hubert Lacey, Christine Craggs-Hinton and Kate Robinson

Overcoming Anxiety
Dr Windy Dryden

Overcoming Depression
Dr Windy Dryden and Sarah Opie

Overcoming Emotional Abuse
Susan Elliot-Wright

Overcoming Hurt
Dr Windy Dryden

Overcoming Insomnia
Susan Elliot-Wright

Overcoming Jealousy
Dr Windy Dryden

Overcoming Panic and Related Anxiety Disorders
Margaret Hawkins

Overcoming Gambling: A guide for problem and compulsive gamblers
Philip Mawer

Overcoming Procrastination
Dr Windy Dryden

Overcoming Shyness and Social Anxiety
Dr Ruth Searle

Overcoming Tiredness and Exhaustion
Fiona Marshall

Reducing Your Risk of Cancer
Dr Terry Priestman

Safe Dieting for Teens
Linda Ojeda

Self-discipline: How to get it and how to keep it
Dr Windy Dryden

The Self-Esteem Journal
Alison Waines

Simplify Your Life
Naomi Saunders

Sinusitis: Steps to healing
Dr Paul Carson

Stammering: Advice for all ages
Renée Byrne and Louise Wright

Stress-related Illness
Dr Tim Cantopher

Ten Steps to Positive Living
Dr Windy Dryden

Think Your Way to Happiness
Dr Windy Dryden and Jack Gordon

Tranquillizers and Antidepressants: When to take them, how to stop
Professor Malcolm Lader

The Traveller's Good Health Guide
Dr Ted Lankester

Treating Arthritis Diet Book
Margaret Hills

Treating Arthritis: The drug-free way
Margaret Hills and Christine Horner

Treating Arthritis: More ways to a drug-free life
Margaret Hills

Understanding Obsessions and Compulsions
Dr Frank Tallis

Understanding Traumatic Stress
Dr Nigel Hunt and Dr Sue McHale

When Someone You Love Has Dementia
Susan Elliot-Wright

When Someone You Love Has Depression
Barbara Baker

Overcoming Common Problems

Motor Neurone Disease

A family affair

Third edition

DR DAVID OLIVER

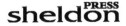

First published in Great Britain in 1995

Sheldon Press
36 Causton Street
London SW1P 4ST
www.sheldonpress.co.uk

Second edition published 2006
Reprinted once
Third edition published 2011

The author and publisher have made every effort to ensure that the
external website and email addresses included in this book are correct and
up to date at the time of going to press. The author and publisher are not
responsible for the content, quality or continuing accessibility of the sites.

British Library Cataloguing-in-Publication Data
A catalogue record for this book is available from the British Library

ISBN 978–1–84709–153–6

1 3 5 7 9 10 8 6 4 2

Typeset by Fakenham Photosetting Ltd, Fakenham, Norfolk
Printed in Great Britain by Ashford Colour Press

Produced on paper from sustainable forests

Author's dedication
This book is dedicated to all those who have motor neurone disease and the carers who help them.

Publisher's dedication
We would like to thank Jeremy Bakewell, our Sales Representative in the Midlands, for the original idea for this book. His father Edgar had motor neurone disease, and sadly died in October 1989. This book is dedicated to him and to Jeremy.

Contents

Foreword by Tricia Holmes   xi

Acknowledgements   xv

Note to the reader   xvi

Introduction   xvii

1 What is motor neurone disease?   1

2 What will the doctor do?   10

3 What treatment can be given?   18

4 How can I cope with motor neurone disease?   22

5 How will my family cope?   35

6 Facing the future   46

7 Who will be caring for me?   62

8 The role of the Motor Neurone Disease Association   74

9 What other help is available?   82

Useful addresses   95

Further reading   101

Index   105

Foreword

Thanks to advances in care and research, we currently know more about motor neurone disease (MND) than we have at any other time. Today we understand more than ever how good-quality care from professionals such as doctors, therapists and nurses makes an enormous difference to the quality of life of someone with the disease. We know that diagnosis can be made more quickly and with more certainty, and that there has never been more information available to those affected by the disease, and the professionals who look after them.

We know all this – but we still don't understand what causes over 90 per cent of cases of MND, or how to cure it. However, what Dr Oliver's book shows is how much can be done to help someone with the disease live their life to the full.

The Motor Neurone Disease Association campaigns to ensure people with MND get the best care available, and that they can make informed choices about that care. Everyone's experience of MND is unique, and so are their needs. It has never been more important for people to understand what options for care, treatment and day-to-day living are open to them, and for their voices to be heard by those who provide this care.

The Motor Neurone Disease Association has developed a benchmark for the level of care we believe everyone living with MND should be able to expect. These 'Standards of Care' are the basis of our ongoing work to educate all those involved in providing care services to people with MND. They set out the needs of people living with MND at three stages: before, at the time of, and following their diagnosis.

People with MND need to receive the right diagnosis quickly and sensitively. In addition, they need to be in contact with a single person – a 'key worker' – who can ensure that all their support and care, no matter who provides it, is properly planned and coordinated. Our role at the Association is to make sure these things happen. The aim of this proactive approach is to help people with MND make informed choices about living with the disease, while at the same time feeling supported and achieving quality of life.

All of the services and support needed to help cope with MND exist through the NHS, local authority social services and the benefits system. But these organizations were not originally set up with a condition like MND in mind. Trying to find out what is available, under what rules, and to coordinate this around the needs of each individual can be an immense burden, both for the patient and the carer.

In 2005 the government published its National Service Framework for Long-term Neurological Conditions, a set of 'quality requirements' that all health and social care providers must adhere to when providing care for people with conditions like MND, Parkinson's disease and Alzheimer's disease. The aim of the Framework is to put the patient at the centre of the network of care that is available, rather than leaving them to navigate their own way around what can be a complicated and bureaucratic healthcare system.

This recognition of the unique needs of people with conditions like MND is a massive step forward, and the Motor Neurone Disease Association will be lobbying at all levels of health and social services to make sure that rapidly progressing conditions like MND are the priority as the Framework is implemented at a local level.

Ensuring people affected by MND receive the care and support they need forms one half of the Motor Neurone Disease Association's mission. Our other objective is to promote and fund research into causes of and treatments for the disease, as well as the search for a cure. While research often turns up exciting new developments, the breakthrough in terms of an effective treatment or cure is sadly still many years away.

Dr Oliver's message is a simple one. For generations it was assumed that nothing could be done about MND. This book shows that the reverse is true: that there is an immense amount that can be done about virtually every aspect of the disease and its symptoms. We know more now than we ever did before about MND – and the fact that our knowledge grows all the time is what keeps our hope alive.

Tricia Holmes
Former Director of Care Development,
Motor Neurone Disease Association

Acknowledgements

I would like to thank the many people who have helped me in the preparation of this book, including the staff at the Wisdom Hospice; other members of the Motor Neurone Disease Clinical Meeting; regional care development advisers; and staff at the Motor Neurone Disease Association; Joyce Onslow, Association visitor for the Mid-Kent Branch; and all who have read earlier drafts and helped me with their comments. I would also like to thank Joanna Moriarty, Rima Devereaux and all at Sheldon Press for their help and advice.

Finally, my thanks go to all the patients and their families who have allowed me to share in their care and have shown me so much.

Note to the reader

This is not a medical book and is not intended to replace advice from your doctor. Consult your pharmacist or doctor if you believe you have any of the symptoms described, and if you think you might need medical help.

Introduction

This book aims to serve as an introduction to and source of information on motor neurone disease. There are only about 5000 people with the disease in the United Kingdom. However, for every affected person, and their family, the reality of the disease can be very frightening. Often fear is worsened by ignorance and misinformation. By providing answers to some of the questions you may have, I hope that it may be a little easier to cope with the effects of the disease and get on with living.

Although there are many common features of motor neurone disease, every person is different and the problems that may develop can vary greatly. In writing a book about a disease that varies from person to person, I am aware that some people may become worried as they read about problems they do not have themselves and have never really thought about. There are problems that may never affect one individual but can be severe for someone else. Unfortunately, the media can increase the fears experienced by people with the disease as the coverage of motor neurone disease often stresses the more difficult and distressing aspects of the disease. These changes are not universal and will not necessarily happen to everyone who has the disease. I hope that by providing information about motor neurone disease and describing the course of the disease, and what may happen as it develops, this book will help to allay fears and give you a more balanced view.

Motor neurone disease affects everyone differently, but often you, and your family, feel rather helpless when you first find out that this is the diagnosis. There may be little support or help given at the time and, as it is an uncommon disease, the doctors and nurses may not be very knowledgeable about it. However, there is much that can be done and many ways in which help can be provided. At the present time there is no cure, but the effects of the disease can be lessened, allowing life to continue as normally as possible. The disease will vary in its effect, the time taken for changes to occur and the help needed, but there is always something more that can be done to help – whether this takes the form of drugs, the provision of helping aids or support and comfort.

I have been closely involved in the care of people with motor neurone disease for over 26 years. It has been a privilege to know and care for them and their families and to share in their experiences of the disease. At the Wisdom Hospice, we care for about 20 people at home at any one time, and a large number of these have been cared for at home until their death. I hope that I have been able to help them to control their symptoms and cope with their problems. I have also been closely involved in the support of the local branch of the Motor Neurone Disease Association, and I am President of the Mid-Kent Branch.

My intention in writing this book has been to create a source of reference that you can dip into and read about the aspects of the disease that are worrying you. Some points and details are repeated in different parts of the book so that all the necessary information on a subject is available to you even if you only read one chapter of the book.

It aims to provide some answers to some of the questions you may wish to ask and, I hope, will show that there is help and support for everyone, however they are affected by motor neurone disease.

1

What is motor neurone disease?

Introduction

Motor neurone disease is a very variable disease that, at present, cannot be cured, although much can be done to ease its effects. Hearing that you, or someone close to you, may have the disease, can be very hard. There may be many feelings at this time, including a sense of shock, depression and fear. I hope that this chapter will explain a little more about the disease and will provide answers to some of the questions on your mind. However, motor neurone disease has such a variety of different effects on different people that everyone with the disease has their own combination of them – each, therefore, having their own particular needs.

The cause of motor neurone disease is not yet known. The main effect of the disease is the damage and death of a specific group of nerve cells called the motor neurones, most of which are in the spinal cord and the base of the brain. These nerve cells control the muscles of the body, and their death means that the muscles can no longer work as usual and become weaker. The extent of the cell damage can be very variable, and so the effects on the muscles can be equally varied.

What is a motor neurone?

A motor neurone is a nerve cell that carries messages from the brain to the muscles of the body. There are two main types of motor neurone cells. The upper motor neurones start in the outer part of the brain and pass down the spinal cord towards the body. The route taken by the nerves is complicated as, in the lowest part of the brain, the nerves cross to the other side and pass down the spinal cord on that side within the part of the spinal cord called the corticospinal tracts. These nerves pass down the spinal cord to the points in the body where they meet the nerves that will pass the messages on to the nerves that act on the muscles (see Figure 1).

The upper motor neurone passes on the message to the lower motor neurone. This nerve passes out of the spinal cord and to the muscle it controls. The message passes across from one nerve to the other at a junction area (called the synapse), and the electrical message transfers from cell to cell by means of a chemical that is released from the upper motor neurone and is passed across to the lower motor neurone.

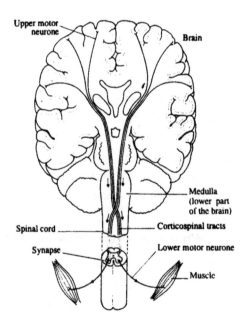

Figure 1 Motor neurones

What happens in motor neurone disease?

When a person develops motor neurone disease, there is damage to these motor neurones. The effects of this damage depend on the type of nerve affected. If the lower motor neurone is affected, the muscle becomes weak and floppy. There are other changes that can be detected, such as a rippling effect under the skin (medically termed fasciculation), which is caused because the different parts of the muscles are no longer properly controlled and start to work independently.

If the upper motor neurones are damaged, the muscles become weak and stiffen. The nerves that go to the muscles of the head and neck area arise from the base of the brain and they may be upper or lower motor neurones. The muscles that are normally controlled by these nerves are then affected, including those involved in the movement of the tongue, in swallowing, in speaking and in the control of the muscles of the face. The effects of this damage can be to cause problems with speech and swallowing and, on occasions, difficulty in controlling the expression of some feelings, leading to unexplained laughter or crying.

Are there different types of motor neurone disease?

All people with motor neurone disease vary in the way that the body is affected. However, there are three main forms of the condition.

- *Amyotrophic lateral sclerosis* This occurs in about two-thirds of patients. With this there is both upper and lower motor neurone damage, so the effects are of stiffness, particularly of the legs, and weakness. This form of the disease is more common in men than women and starts later in life, usually when the person is over 55 years old.
- *Progressive bulbar palsy* This occurs in about a quarter of people

with the disease. There is lower motor neurone damage of the nerves to the head and neck. In this form of the disease there are problems with swallowing and speech.

- *Progressive muscular atrophy* This accounts for only about one in ten of all who develop the condition and is much more common in men than women (of the people affected by this form of motor neurone disease, 80 per cent are men). It starts at an earlier age than the other forms, in people under 50 years old. In this form, there are signs of lower motor nerve loss and there is weakness and wasting of muscles, especially in the arms.

Although these forms of motor neurone disease are described in the textbooks, and a doctor may give a name to the form of the disease, as there is often a mixture of effects depending on the exact combination of nerves damaged, it is not always possible to give a clear name to the type of motor neurone disease a person has. As a person becomes more ill, there is a further nerve loss and all of the features of the disease are mixed. It is important to stress that all the features of the condition may or may not occur as everyone is so different.

Certain problems, though, seem to be rare in motor neurone disease. Loss of control of the bladder and bowels is rare, for example, and there is not often any change in touch and the other senses. Changes in the brain itself, causing confusion or loss of other mental functions, are also rare and affect fewer than one person in ten.

How common is motor neurone disease?

Approximately one in every 50 000 people develop motor neurone disease each year, so about 1100 people are found to have the disease in the UK every year. At any time, there are between 5000 and 6000 people in the UK with the disease. It is not a common disease, but as it often progresses over a period of three to four years, there are actually more people dying from motor neurone disease every year than from other more common diseases, such as multiple sclerosis.

Who is affected by motor neurone disease?

At the moment, there is no known cause of motor neurone disease, and so it is not clear why a particular person develops it. Men in middle to old age seem to be affected more commonly than women, and the average age when the disease is diagnosed is about 56, although it is also found in younger people. If there is a family history of the disease, the average age at diagnosis is younger – 53 – and again, men are more often affected than women. There are many theories as to the cause of the disease, but there does not appear to be any connection with social class, activity or diet.

Is motor neurone disease becoming more common?

There is evidence that motor neurone disease is being found more often. During the last 30 years, the number of people diagnosed with the condition in England and Wales has nearly doubled, whereas the number of people found to have multiple sclerosis has stayed constant.

This increase may be partly due to more accurate testing and diagnosis. There is also evidence that motor neurone disease is more common in the elderly and, as the number of older people increases in the general population, so the condition will become more common.

What are the effects in the early stages?

The early effects of motor neurone disease are often very slight and develop gradually. For nine out of ten people, there is a slow and gradual increase in weakness, and the area most affected will depend on which nerves are damaged.

Clumsiness and weakness of the hands develops in the early stages of progressive muscular atrophy, and there may be difficulty in using the fingers, such as in writing or doing up buttons or zips.

Tripping and problems with walking may be the first signs with the form of motor neurone disease known as amyotrophic lateral sclerosis. Difficulties may be experienced climbing or going down stairs, or the person may trip easily, particularly on the edges of pavements or on uneven ground. This can be a cause of embarrassment as a person having difficulty walking may even be thought by others to be drunk.

Some people first notice the changes in the muscles, such as the rippling of muscles under the skin when the lower motor nerves have been damaged (the fasciculation mentioned earlier) or the wasting and thinning of muscles. Others may develop cramp as the muscles become stiff.

Slurred speech or difficulty in swallowing may be the first evidence of progressive bulbar palsy. These changes may be slight at first and develop slowly, so that the person affected may be unaware of the early changes. However, others may notice the slurring and even ask if the person is drunk.

Breathing problems are rare in the early stages of motor neurone disease, but occasionally, if the muscles involved in breathing become weakened, the first manifestations of the condition may be breathlessness. Rarely, the disease may only be recognized when breathing problems develop after an operation and artificial ventilation has been required to help the person breathe.

Every person will develop the disease in a different way, and there are no hard and fast rules with motor neurone disease. When all people with the disease are considered together, about four in every ten people notice the first changes in the arms and hands, four in ten notice the changes in the legs, and two in ten first develop changes in speech or swallowing.

What causes motor neurone disease?

Since the French neurologist Jean-Martin Charcot described the disease in 1874, there have been many theories as to the cause. However, no theory has stood the test of time, although there is increasing research into the changes in the spinal cord and the effects of the disease.

About one in 20 people with motor neurone disease has a family history of the disease, and there appears to be at least one form of the disease that is, in fact, hereditary. It seems that this form occurs when there is an altered area in the genetic code that is passed on from parent to child. This pattern of inheritance is described as autosomal dominance, and the affected code is passed from the parent to one in two of the children and, if this code is present, the child may develop the disease.

Recent research has shown that in one form of motor neurone disease, the defective gene (part of the genetic message) is on one particular chromosome in the cell – chromosome 21. This gene (SOD1) is involved in the production of an enzyme called superoxide dismutase. Other abnormal genes, or mutations, have also been found on other chromosomes.

It is not clear at present how the abnormal gene affects nerve cells. It is thought that the abnormal proteins that are produced by these abnormal genes damage the structure of the cell and other proteins, leading to the cell's death.

Although this research may herald a possibility of finding out more about the cause of the disease, there may also be ethical dilemmas. It may be possible, when the hereditary form of the disease is suspected, to test whole families for the presence of the gene and thus find out if an individual is likely to develop the disease later in life, even if the person shows no signs of the disease at the time. However, finding this out would bring with it a great burden and many worries for all concerned as, at present, there is no cure for the disease.

This new evidence may be the start of a new understanding of the cause of motor neurone disease since other factors, such as chemicals introduced into the body from outside, could also affect and damage enzymes. These could then lead to the damage and later death of the nerve cell. However, these theories are, at present, in a very early stage of development.

Evidence for a dietary cause of the disease has been suggested for one specific area – the island of Guam in the western Pacific Ocean. In the 1950s and 1960s there was on Guam a very high incidence of motor neurone disease, associated with Parkinson's disease and dementia. In the past it was thought that this was caused by the people of this island eating flour made from the cycad plant (false sago palm), which contains a poison. When this poison was extracted from the cycad plant and fed to monkeys, symptoms similar to MND were noticed. However, the situation seems to be more complicated than this, and recent research has shown that the poison is actually passed on to humans through their eating the flying fox fruit bat, a local delicacy. The flying fox fruit bat is able to eat the toxic cycad plant without being harmed, and the poison becomes concentrated within its body. But when the fruit bat is eaten by humans, the poison causes this specific form of MND. When the flying fox fruit bat became rare, the incidence of disease reduced – and it is now no longer seen on the island.

There have been many other theories as to the possible causes. Many different substances have been suggested as leading to the disease, including an excess of heavy metals, such as lead, mercury, manganese or calcium, or a shortage of the metal cobalt. There have also been suggestions that there is an increased risk of the condition in people who have worked in the leather industry and have been in contact with the solvents used in that industry. These theories have never been proved and it seems unlikely that a single substance leads to the development of motor neurone disease.

Viral infection has also been suggested as a cause of the disease. In particular, there was some evidence that motor neurone disease occurred more often in areas of the country where poliomyelitis had been common during the 1950s and 1960s. It was suggested that people may have been infected with the polio virus and that this caused some damage to the nerves, but it did not become apparent until later in life.

Infection by a 'slow virus' has also been suggested. This virus may be contracted early in life but then develops its symptoms slowly, so that the disease is only seen later in life. This has never been confirmed.

Although many theories have been suggested, none has been confirmed over time, so that the cause of motor neurone disease still eludes researchers. There would seem to be a common thread running through these ideas, however, in that there is a period of delay after the initial damage to the body has taken place before the disease develops. Nerve damage may have occurred earlier in life, maybe even caused by one of the factors mentioned, but this damage does not have any great effect at the time and remains unnoticed. As the person becomes older and other nerves die as part of the ageing process, only then do the symptoms of the disease become apparent.

All these theories, though, are unproven at the present time, and research continues. It may be very difficult for you to face a disease that is only partly understood. Often people feel that something or someone, including themselves, is to blame for the disease. These feelings are understandable but, at the moment, there is no evidence that something you have done has caused the disease. It is important to share any such concerns and feelings you may have, especially with those close to you, so that you can all face the disease together without blame and misunderstanding.

2

What will the doctor do?

Introduction

Motor neurone disease is uncommon and often it is difficult for the diagnosis to be made. You may have problems for some time before you have tests that confirm that what you have is motor neurone disease. This will usually involve seeing a hospital specialist in neurology (the medical care of diseases of the nervous system) as well as other medical and nursing professionals.

What happens when I first notice the changes?

The first changes as a result of motor neurone disease may be slight, such as clumsiness when using your hands, tripping or weakness of the legs or slurring of the speech or difficulty in swallowing. At first, these changes may not seem bad enough to see a doctor about. As the changes and problems become worse, though, you will usually see your own GP, who will want to undertake a fuller examination.

The early changes are often vague and may be confused with one of several other diseases. It may be very difficult to make a firm diagnosis in these early stages and other tests may be necessary, such as X-rays to check for arthritis, as this could affect the nerves and cause similar problems. The doctor may not be able to make a diagnosis immediately and may wait to see if there are further changes before referring you on to a specialist.

If the problems continue, you are likely to be referred to a consultant at the hospital for further tests. You will normally see a consultant neurologist, but the specialist could be a general physician, a rheumatologist (who is involved in the care of people with bone, joint and muscle complaints) or a consultant in rehabilitation medicine (who helps people with disability to adapt and cope with this). Usually if you see other specialists, they will refer you on to a neurologist to make the final diagnosis.

What will the doctor do?

The neurologist, or other hospital specialist, will first need you to describe the problems you are experiencing as fully as you can in order to assess the condition as accurately as possible. The doctor will then need to examine you, and the information gained will help the doctor to work out exactly what is wrong. The specialist may then have a good idea as to what the diagnosis should be and may be able to tell you what thoughts he or she has. However, at this early stage the doctor may want to wait until the diagnosis is certain before saying anything one way or the other. Diagnosing someone as having motor neurone disease has many great implications, and so it is only right that there should be conclusive evidence before a person is told that this is the diagnosis.

What tests will be done?

There are several tests that can be done to confirm the diagnosis or to rule out other diseases that can be confused with motor neurone disease. These tests may include the following.

- *A blood test for creatine kinase* A small sample of blood is taken and sent to the laboratory for analysis. Creatine kinase is an enzyme found within the muscles, and a raised level of this enzyme often, but not always, occurs in people with motor neurone disease.

- *MRI (magnetic resonance imaging) scan of the spine and brain* This is a specialized test that can show the nerves and brain clearly. Any pressure on the nerves of the spinal cord from damage to the vertebrae (the bones of the spinal column) or the discs between the vertebrae or changes in the brain will be shown in this scan.

- *Electromyography* This is an electrical test of the muscle and nerves, also known, for short, as EMG. A nerve near the elbow is stimulated with a small electric pulse and a small metal plate, placed over the muscle in the arm, records when the message reaches the muscle. With motor neurone disease, the result is usually normal, as any nerves that have not been damaged work normally, passing the electrical message along the nerve to the muscle. Also, a small needle can be put into the muscle, in the arm or leg, and this records the electrical activity of the muscle. With motor neurone disease, the results of this test are abnormal as the muscle is no longer being completely controlled by the nerves. This test is often used to confirm an initial diagnosis either way.

- *A lumbar puncture* This involves taking a small sample of the fluid that surrounds the spinal cord. This sample can be taken either as an out-patient or in-patient in hospital. You lie down on your side and a small area of skin over the lower back is made numb by means of an injection of local anaesthetic. A needle is gently inserted through the skin until the outer covering of the spinal cord is reached. A few drops of the spinal fluid can then be removed. Usually only a little discomfort is felt during the test but, occasionally, people develop a headache afterwards. It is necessary to rest for a few hours afterwards to reduce the risk of this occurring.

  The fluid is then sent to a laboratory for examination and testing. There are not normally any changes in the spinal fluid with motor neurone disease. Other diseases that cause problems similar to those of the disease do cause changes in the fluid, though, and it is often important to check whether or not these diseases are present.

- *A muscle biopsy* Occasionally it may be necessary to perform this test, which involves removing a small sample of muscle. This is a simple test, and the area of skin over an affected muscle is numbed by injecting a local anaesthetic. A small cut is made into the skin so that a sample of muscle can then be taken and examined in the laboratory. Certain other diseases that are similar to motor neurone disease cause abnormal changes in the muscles, and carrying out a biopsy test allows these to be found or crossed off the list of suspected causes of the person's symptoms.

- *A brain scan* Other tests may be necessary, including a brain scan (also known as a CT or CAT scan) to check for any abnormalities in the brain.

Whom will I see?

Many different people may be involved in carrying out these tests and all their roles are explained in more detail in Chapter 7. There are variations in how different areas and hospitals carry out the tests or what tests they can offer, depending on their facilities and the experience and interests of their doctors.

The diagnosis will often be made during a short stay in hospital, often in a neurology ward, or neurology centre, where the necessary tests can all be carried out by a specialized team within a few days. However, in some areas it may be possible to carry out the tests in a day and then admission to hospital may not be necessary.

The various people who may be involved in your care and in carrying out the tests include the following.

- *Your GP* Your family doctor will have started the tests and referred you to a specialist for further tests. He or she will remain the main doctor caring for you at home, and should have been informed by the specialist of the results of your tests. Your GP can provide you with information about the disease and can be called on by you and your family for help and advice if there are problems. Other members of the primary healthcare team, such as the community (district) nurse, may also be able to help.

- *A neurologist* This is a specialist doctor who sees people who have diseases of the nervous system. This doctor will usually be based in a hospital.

- *A consultant in rehabilitation medicine* This is a specialist doctor who is involved in the care of patients with illnesses that cause, or could cause, disability. He or she may be able to assess your particular needs and provide practical help, such as equipment like wheelchairs.

- *A counsellor or social worker* At many neurology centres, there is a specialist counsellor, nurse or social worker who is available for patients and their families. At the time of the tests, it may be helpful to have an opportunity to talk to a counsellor about some of your concerns. Often the counsellor will be available on the ward or in the out-patient clinic when the doctor tells you more about the results of the tests and the possible diagnosis.

- *Motor Neurone Disease Association regional care development adviser* The Motor Neurone Disease Association provides help and support to people with motor neurone disease (see Chapter 8 for further information). There are regional care development advisers in all parts of the country who are able to visit and explain more about the disease and provide support.

- *A physiotherapist* If there is weakness of the muscles, a physiotherapist can provide help and advice, allowing the most to be made of the strength you still have in your muscles.

- *An occupational therapist* Advice on extra help and aids to help with everyday activities can be provided by an occupational therapist. An assessment of what equipment you might need and things you can do to help yourself may be helpful after the diagnosis has been made.

● *A speech and language therapist* If speech or the ability to swallow are affected, a speech and language therapist can provide help and advice.

In some areas, the first assessment of your situation is made by a team of professionals, including the various experts mentioned above. A team approach allows all the therapists to see you and a treatment plan to be organized. You and your family are included in these plans, and a key worker is chosen who can coordinate all the help that will be provided. The key worker may be any one of the professionals involved in your care, and would usually be the person who is most involved with this and closest to you. Unfortunately, this ideal is not always achieved and then you have to make these arrangements yourself. By reading this book you should be able to find out how to ensure that the care you receive is as good as possible.

What will the doctor say?

After all the tests have been completed, the specialist should see you and your family to give an explanation of the results. The giving of such a diagnosis is never easy and some doctors find it particularly difficult, so it may be necessary to insist on seeing the specialist and press for the details of the diagnosis.

The specialist will be able to give you details of the disease and the exact diagnosis. However, no one can say what will definitely happen as the disease progresses – every person's experience is different. The specialist may be able to answer some of the questions that you wish to ask. Although the specialist should try to answer your questions honestly, he or she may not be able to answer all your queries because the disease does vary so greatly. The specialist will try to judge the best way in which to give you the news of your diagnosis and how you will react to it, but may not always get this completely right. You should feel able to go back to your specialist for a further interview at a later date if you and your family feel that this would be helpful.

It is important to be honest about the diagnosis and to let other family members know. It is helpful if a family member, particularly your partner, is able to attend the appointment with the specialist so that the information is given to you together. If the appointment with the specialist does not allow for all your questions to be answered or there are areas of confusion, it is always possible to approach your GP, who should have been informed of the diagnosis by the specialist.

What do I tell my family?

When facing a diagnosis of motor neurone disease, it is usually best that a family shares this knowledge honestly. Naturally, there may be a time of distress and sadness, but this is prefer-able to the anxieties and problems that can occur if the truth is not shared. If one member of the family learns more of the truth than the others, this becomes a large, and often intoler-able, burden for that person. Within a family, the concerns and worries are often apparent, however carefully everyone tries to behave as normally as possible.

Many people, on first hearing the bad news, want to try to protect those who are close to them from it. However, the fam-ily's anxiety may actually increase in this situation, as the worry and effort to conceal the hurt are sensed but not expressed. Sharing the news together allows everyone to express their feel-ings and prevents barriers developing within the family.

What do I do now?

There may be a need to ask further questions and to talk more about the diagnosis with your doctor and with your family.

It would normally be possible to arrange to see the specialist again after a short period so that the many further questions that come to mind can be answered. If this is not possible, you may be able to discuss the situation with your GP, but it may be necessary to allow a short time to elapse so that any letters from the specialist will have had time to reach the doctor's surgery.

There are other sources of information that can be helpful at this time, including the Motor Neurone Disease Association (see Chapter 8 for details and for the number of their helpline). Details of local groups may be available from the hospital, the out-patient clinic or neurological ward, your GP's surgery or a local library or Citizens' Advice Bureau.

If there are important questions that you feel you need answered, ask, and keep on asking, until you feel that they have been answered to your satisfaction. However, always remember that there are some questions that can never be completely answered because the disease is so variable in its effects and no one can look into the future and predict exactly what is going to happen in your case. All that can be expected is that as clear an answer as possible is given, with an explanation of the possible outcomes and options.

3

What treatment can be given?

Introduction

Many treatments for motor neurone disease have been suggested, but research has not confirmed whether or not any of them is effective. However, new treatments are being tested all the time and you may be offered the chance to take part in a trial of a new treatment.

What is a drug trial?

Any new drug is first tested on animals to check for any obvious side-effects and it is then given to healthy volunteers to see if it is safe in humans. It is then necessary to try the drug on people with the disease to check if it has any side-effects in them. The drug is then tested on more patients to see if it is effective in either controlling or reversing the disease. This process is called a clinical trial.

The new drug is compared to either an existing treatment or a dummy treatment, or placebo. Some patients are given the new treatment and some are given the existing treatment or the placebo, but neither the patient nor the doctors most closely involved in the trial know which patient receives which. After a period of time, the length of which depends on the treatment, the two groups of patients are compared and it is revealed which received the new treatment. Only then can the effectiveness or otherwise of the new treatment be assessed and the side-effects, if any, be shown to be acceptable.

If a placebo treatment is not used, a new treatment may

appear to be helpful, but this could just be chance. A new treatment could then look as if it were helpful and this would not necessarily be so, which would lead to many patients in the future receiving a useless, or even harmful, treatment.

Before patients are included in a clinical trial, they have to undergo a full assessment and examination. For the trial to be successful, it is necessary to choose patients who are similar in terms of symptoms, age, length of time since diagnosis and rate of progression, as far as this can be estimated. As a result, not everyone who applies to take part may be included in a clinical trial. Indeed, you may not be included in the trial, even after undergoing all the preliminary tests, because you do not fit the chosen criteria. It is often helpful to discuss all the tests with the doctors involved in the trial before starting on any of them, so that you are aware of the possibilities and the implications of taking part in the trial. You may also wish to discuss the assessments that it will be necessary for you to undergo while you take part, and whether or not they will be undertaken in a centre, perhaps a long way from your home, or be arranged more locally. If you would need to travel long distances, you may feel that the risk of becoming very tired and the burden of the travelling on you and your family are too great. It may be possible to receive financial help with the travelling costs, however. You also need to be aware that you may receive the placebo (dummy) medication, and you and your family need to discuss how you feel about taking part in a trial when you may never receive real medication. There is also the possibility that you could experience side-effects if you do actually receive the medication.

Involvement in such a research project can be both tiring and time-consuming. However, it is only by carrying out such trials of treatment that any progress in the long-term aim of finding a cure for motor neurone disease will be made. You may feel that taking part in a trial will at least be your way of doing something in the search for a treatment and possible cure for motor neurone disease. Research *is* necessary and many patients do feel that it is useful to take part in it, both for themselves and those people who will develop the disease in the future.

What has research shown so far?

During 1994 two large trials of treatments for motor neurone disease reported their results. A large European trial of branched chain amino acids showed that those who took part did not seem to benefit at all from this treatment.

In 1994 the ALS/Riluzole Study Group published the results of a large trial of a new drug, riluzole, in the *New England Journal of Medicine*. Riluzole alters the action of a substance called gluta-mate in the brain. Glutamate is used by nerve cells, including motor nerve cells, for transmitting messages from one nerve cell to another – hence it is known as a transmitter. It has been suggested that glutamate may become overactive in the brain and spinal cord of people with motor neurone disease, causing nerve damage. It is thought that riluzole reduces the effect of glutamate and slows down the changes caused by the disease.

The trials have shown that people taking riluzole live longer than did those taking the placebo medication. This has now been accepted by the National Institute for Health and Clinical Excellence (NICE), and riluzole can now be prescribed for anyone with the definite amyotrophic lateral sclerosis form of the disease. The medication should be started by a neurologist with experi-ence in the care of people with MND, and it is necessary to have regular blood tests, to check that there are no changes in the blood count or functioning of the liver. This is not yet a *cure* for the disease, but it is a start in the search for better treatments.

There have been many trials of other medications over the last few years but, as yet, no new medication has been found that has an appreciable effect on MND. There are other trials being planned though, and further details of these can be obtained from your neurology centre or the Motor Neurone Disease Association (see page 99 for their address).

The use of stem cells is also being investigated. Stem cells are obtained from human embryos or from the bone marrow of adults. These cells have the ability to develop into any type of cell, and it is thought that they could be encouraged to develop into nerve cells in the body. There has been early research in this field, and there are some indications in the laboratory that this may be possible. However, there is no clear evidence as yet that stem cells can be used in the treatment of MND. Research is continuing and it is hoped that this will be helpful.

Although there is no definite indication that the use of stem cells would be beneficial, there are doctors in certain centres across the world who are offering 'treatment'. Stem cells are injected into the blood or spinal fluid in the hope that they will develop within the body, replace damaged cells, and so allow the nerves, and then the muscles, to work again. To repeat, there is no evidence that this treatment is helpful at the present time, and there is still a need for research to ensure that such treatment is not potentially harmful.

The use of vitamin C and vitamin E has been suggested as a possible treatment. These vitamins help to reduce free radicals in the body. As it has been suggested that the formation of free radicals may be involved in causing motor neurone disease, a medication that reduces their presence in the cells may be of help. As yet, though, the effectiveness of these vitamins has not been proved.

Many other treatments for motor neurone disease have been tried and some doctors may suggest the use of these, such as vitamin B12 injections, but there is no evidence that they are effective. If you are unsure about the treatment that has been suggested, discuss this with your neurologist or GP. If you are unhappy about the advice you receive, you may wish to discuss the possibility of getting a second opinion.

4

How can I cope with motor neurone disease?

Introduction

Although, at the time of writing, there is no treatment that will cure motor neurone disease, there is a great deal that can be done to relieve or cope with some of the symptoms. There are many symptoms that may occur with the disease, but you will not experience all of them. Also, how you will be affected will be different from how anyone else will be affected. In discussing the problems that may occur, I am aware that a frightening list begins to form. However, it is necessary to consider all instances and to stress that whatever does develop, there are ways of coping with it to allow you to have as full a life as possible.

The various symptoms are considered separately, together with the treatments available.

Will there be any pain?

Pain may occur with motor neurone disease, even though the nerves that sense pain are not directly affected by the disease. When the muscles become weaker, there may be pain in the joints – in particular the shoulder joint, as there is then greater strain on this joint. This pain can be eased by taking a bone pain relief tablet, such as ketoprofen or naproxen or, on occasion, by having an injection of local anaesthetic into the joint.

Muscles that become stiff because of the disease may develop painful cramps. Taking regular exercise and the advice of a physiotherapist can be helpful and, on occasions, muscle relaxant tablets, such as baclofen or dantrolene, may be suggested. A physiotherapist may also be able to show you and your carer how to move your limbs to ease the stiffness in your joints and muscles.

Pain may also be felt as a result of having to stay in the same position for some time if, say, it becomes difficult to move. Being helped to change position regularly may be all that is needed, but if the discomfort becomes worse, painkillers may be needed. Sometimes the regular use of simple painkillers, such as paracetamol or co-codamol, may be sufficient. However, often stronger painkillers, such as morphine as a liquid medicine or tablets, may be necessary. Morphine can cause nausea in some people when it is first taken and an anti-sickness medicine, such as prochlorperazine, haloperidol or domperidone, may need to be taken for the first few days. Constipation may also be a side-effect and then laxatives may be necessary.

Many people, often including doctors, worry about the use of morphine to treat people as they fear the patient will become addicted or its use will shorten their life. *Any* medicine is potentially dangerous if misused. Morphine can be dangerous if it is misused, but in the control of pain, the drug may be used safely, with few side-effects. People have taken morphine medicines for months, or even years, without any harmful effects, and have experienced much better control of their discomfort and pain than with other forms of medication. If you have any concerns about the medicines, discuss them with your doctor or nurse.

Will I become breathless?

Some people with motor neurone disease do feel more short of breath as the muscles of the chest that are involved in breathing become weaker. If it does occur, it may be noticed first as shortness of breath when you are more active, such as walking upstairs or uphill. If the muscles weaken still more, breathing may even be short while sitting and resting. A cough may also be noticed, particularly together with a need to clear the throat, and this may occur when there are breathing problems.

A physiotherapist may be helpful as he or she can advise on breathing exercises you can do and ensure that your posture is such that it allows for as much expansion of the chest as possible. Antibiotics may be necessary if there is marked breathlessness and the need to cough, and relaxants, such as diazepam, may be helpful in relaxing the muscles of the chest and reducing the feelings of breathlessness.

If the feelings of shortness of breath become more troublesome, morphine medication may be suggested. Morphine can be very helpful, relieving the breathlessness and allowing greater activity. Sometimes the weakness of the breathing muscles can cause other problems, and help may be needed to support breathing – such as non-invasive ventilation (see pages 48–9).

What happens if I have problems swallowing?

If the nerves to the head and neck are affected by the disease, the muscles of the mouth and throat may become weaker and swallowing may become more difficult. At first, swallowing may just feel different, but it may worsen so that it becomes difficult to swallow food and drink.

There are many ways in which you can help yourself to swallow better. A speech and language therapist can advise you on how to do this, and a dietitian can tell you about suitable foods and supplementary foods that can be taken (see page 70). It may be necessary to experiment to find foods or drinks that are easier to take. For instance, many people find that 'soft solids', such as soups, custards, jellies and moist foods, are easier to swallow than drinks or dry foods. It is important to take time over meals and not to rush your eating. A heated food tray may be helpful as then your food will stay appetizingly hot, even if you eat the meal slowly. It is also important that you are sitting upright with your head level and supported. Some people find it helps to have an iced drink or suck an ice cube before eating. The Motor Neurone Disease Association produces a very helpful leaflet concerning problems with swallowing, with advice on diet.

What can I do if I dribble?

If swallowing does become more difficult, it may also become difficult to swallow the saliva you produce. As every person is different, though, this problem is not experienced by all people with motor neurone disease.

Every day, the average person forms up to 1 litre (2 pints) of saliva, and a person with motor neurone disease also produces this amount. If swallowing becomes difficult, it may not be possible for you to swallow all the saliva you produce and it may dribble out of your mouth. This is obviously very distressing as we tend to associate dribbling with babyhood or people with other handicaps. On occasion, other people can think that a person dribbling has mental problems. It is important to explain the cause of the problem to others so that they can understand and accept it.

It is possible to use medication to reduce the amount of saliva formed. These drugs can, however, make the mouth feel too dry and it is necessary to use them very carefully and find the correct dose. The drugs include atropine (available as a tablet or liquid) and hyoscine.

Hyoscine can be given as a tablet that dissolves under the tongue, and is available from pharmacists as the seasickness tablet Kwells. These tablets can be helpful and, as they act quickly and for only a few hours, they can be taken before the saliva becomes too troublesome, such as at night to reduce the saliva problems while you are asleep. Hyoscine is also available as a patch that releases the medication slowly into the body through the skin, which is very useful if swallowing is difficult, or as an injection if the problem becomes much worse.

If you prefer not to use drugs, a portable suction pump can be useful to remove excess saliva from your mouth (the Motor Neurone Disease Association can provide this equipment if necessary).

What is meant by tube feeding?

For some, but by no means all, swallowing may become so difficult that it becomes impossible to take in enough food in the usual way to maintain a normal weight. Eating may gradually become more difficult so that meals take longer and longer. Then, alternative methods of feeding may need to be considered, and discussion with, and advice from, a speech and language therapist and dietitian will be helpful.

If you have seen these specialists regularly during your illness, they can monitor your swallowing and advise you as to what would be the most suitable way of coping with the problem should it occur. One way in which you can be helped is by the insertion of a small feeding tube through the stomach wall, so that food can be fed directly into the stomach. This is known as a percutaneous endoscopic gastrostomy (PEG; see pages 50–1).

What can be done for speech problems?

Many people, but not all, develop problems with speech if the nerves to the muscles of the head and neck are affected. This may start as a slurring of speech. Others may think that you are drunk, but it is important to ensure that people you meet understand that the speech difficulties are, in fact, due to motor neurone disease.

If problems with speech worsen, it may become increasingly difficult to be understood and other ways of communicating may be necessary. It is helpful to keep sentences short and to the point – even if this goes against the grain and seems impolite – as it allows the important part of the message to be spoken before the muscles become tired. It may also be helpful to start a 'yes and no' signalling system. For instance, particular parts of the body could be moved to signal 'yes' and 'no', such as blinking, a head movement or raising an eyebrow once for 'yes', twice for 'no'. In this way, simple questions can be answered without exertion, as long as they *can* be answered with just a 'yes' or 'no'.

Using a notepad and pencil can be a way of ensuring that your needs are understood. However, there is other equipment that can be helpful, especially if your hands are weaker and writing is difficult.

The advice of a speech and language therapist can be very helpful when speech is starting to become difficult. At this time, the therapist can discuss the various options and allow you to practise on some of the equipment. There is a wide range of equipment available, including spelling boards, which allow you to spell out words, and simple electronic keyboards that write out short sentences that can be seen by both the writer and the listener (Lightwriters). There are also more complicated systems that may be of help. The most sophisticated are connected to computers and allow you to write longer sentences and have certain well-used phrases available within the computer's memory so that they can be printed at the touch of a button. Certain systems can have an artificial voice generator so that you can not only type a message, but the computer can speak it for you too.

Many people find that they can continue to communicate with their family and friends using text messaging on their mobile phones. Increasingly, the use of computers and email allows communication to continue, even if speech is affected.

These more sophisticated communication aids are not widely available, but a speech and language therapist can advise you as to what aid would be best for you and what is available in your area. There are some communication aids centres around the UK where you can be carefully assessed and have the opportunity to try out some of the aids.

Can I use a telephone?

One important form of communication in everyday life is the telephone, but if it becomes harder and harder to speak, it will become increasingly difficult to talk to family and friends on the phone and even to call for help in an emergency. It is possible to use a kind of Morse code, tapping on the mouthpiece, to communicate some basic information, but the conversation will become rather one-sided. There are telephones that can be programmed with certain words or phrases that allow some two-way conversation. The Typetalk communication system, operated by the Royal National Institute for Deaf People, may also allow you to use the telephone more easily. With this, you can type your message on a special type of telephone and a Typetalk operator speaks your message to your caller, who can speak their message back to you.

An answerphone can be helpful as it allows other people to telephone you and leave a message without your having to answer the telephone. Many answerphones also allow the caller to speak by way of a loudspeaker, which may make it easier for you to use a phone if your arms are weak.

How can I call for help?

It is important to ensure that help can be sought in an emergency. In the house, a buzzer system can allow you to attract the attention of others, although if hand movements are restricted, a special sensitive switch may be needed so that it can be operated by just a small movement. Otherwise, the telephone can be used to summon help, if you can dial the number and then use a prearranged code of taps. There are also telephone systems that allow help to be summoned simply by pressing an alarm, which can be kept on a necklace or attached to clothing.

How can I stay independent?

There are also more complicated systems that can be used to help with communication, and to control what is going on around you. For example, a small movement of a hand, leg or head, or using the suck/blow tube of an electronic system, can be used to type on a display screen, activate an artificial voice, operate a door-opening switch or put on a switch, allowing the television to be controlled or the light to be turned on or off. These systems can help you to be more independent as well as to communicate with others. A speech and language therapist, occupational therapist or a disablement services centre can advise you on how suitable these systems are for you and how to use them.

What happens if walking is difficult?

If the muscles in the legs weaken, walking may become difficult. At first, this may only be felt on occasions, say tripping when the feet are not lifted up properly and the toes catch on the ground. Later the weakness may be felt when walking medium to longer distances or climbing stairs.

Although no treatment can make the muscles stronger once the nerves to these muscles have been damaged by the disease, exercise may allow the most to be made of the strength that the muscles still have. A physiotherapist can assess the strength of various muscles and show you exercises to do to maintain as much movement as possible. Doing exercises will also help to stop the muscles becoming stiff and so help keep you feeling comfortable.

It may be helpful to use a walking stick or frame to reduce the risks of you falling (they help to keep the body balanced and give support). If the legs become even weaker, it may be necessary to consider using a wheelchair. Many people try to avoid using a wheelchair as they feel that this will be 'giving in' to the illness and are frightened that other people will treat them differently if they do so. Although there are problems associated with using a wheelchair, as many places have restricted access, there are also benefits. If the amount of energy and strength you have is less than it used to be, a wheelchair allows longer distances to be covered quickly and easily, allowing you to save your energy for walking yourself at the more important times. An occupational therapist, a wheelchair clinic or a disablement services centre will be able to advise you on the correct choice in your circumstances.

Putting off using a wheelchair until it is really necessary can cause unnecessary problems. It will usually take time – sometimes up to a few weeks – for a chair to be ordered and delivered, and so it is helpful to make the order well before it is necessary. It may at first only be used on rare occasions, such as when you want to go out with members of the family or friends and this will involve walking further than you are able to, but at least you will have it when you need it.

Other help may also be necessary as walking and moving about becomes more difficult. Getting up out of a chair, for example, can be a struggle, but there are specialized aids to help with this. Electrically powered chairs that can slowly raise you to a standing position, for example, make life much easier. Again, your occupational therapist will be able to advise you on what is available.

Can I help my stiff muscles?

If the nerves damaged by the disease are mainly the upper motor neurones (see pages 1–3), the muscles may become stiffer than normal. This may feel uncomfortable and make it more difficult to move about. It is important to make sure that the arms and legs are in the best possible position to do whatever activity you have planned, so that the muscles are as relaxed as possible. Exercising regularly can also be very helpful, and a physiotherapist can provide advice on the best exercises. There is medication that can help to relax muscles, such as tizanidine, baclofen and diazepam, but they all need to be used with care as they can have some side-effects if the dose is increased too quickly. These medicines can also be helpful if you experience cramps in the stiff muscles, and quinine sulphate may also be used. Your doctor and nurse can discuss the use of these drugs with you.

What can I do if I cannot sleep?

There are many reasons for not being able to sleep. Sometimes the main problem is discomfort or pain when you are lying in bed, especially if, because of weakness, it is difficult to turn and adjust your position. Careful positioning when settling at night and regular changes of position may help you have a more comfortable night, but on occasions, painkillers may be helpful. Morphine, taken in liquid or tablet form, may be particularly helpful (see page 23).

Some people find that they cannot sleep because they are concerned that they may not be able to call for help in the night as they have difficulty speaking. It can help to put the mind at rest by having a buzzer fitted so that this can be used to attract the attention of others in the house when necessary. This can have a sensitive switch, which can be operated by only a small movement of a hand or leg.

On occasions, taking a sleeping tablet may be helpful, such as temazepam or diazepam. Many people try to avoid taking sleeping tablets, but they can be very helpful in getting a good night's sleep, allowing the days to be enjoyed and not marred by tiredness. Many sleeping tablets can also have the effect of relaxing stiff muscles and so may help to reduce discomfort and cramps.

What about my bowels?

When eating is more difficult and you are less active, the bowels may become more sluggish. It is important to make sure that you include a good amount of roughage in your diet and have plenty of drinks. Even if little is eaten or the food you have at any one point is low in roughage, bowel movements should still be regular. Many people think that as the diet is reduced, the bowels will stop functioning altogether, but if the bowels are ignored, much discomfort and distress may occur as constipation worsens. On occasion, laxatives may be necessary, but their use should be supervised by your doctor or nurse so that the best combination for your needs is used. Rarely, suppositories and enemas may be needed, but if you look after your bowels, this is less likely to be necessary.

Will I have problems passing water?

As we saw in Chapter 1, motor neurone disease does not affect the control of the bladder or bowels. However, you may find it a little more difficult to pass urine if the muscles of the abdomen become weak. If walking and moving are difficult, it may be difficult physically to get to a toilet, and then extra help may be needed to make sure that you are able to reach the toilet when you want to. Only rarely is a catheter (a tube inserted into the bladder to drain the water into a bag) necessary.

Will I get bed sores?

Anyone who stays in one position for a long time may develop a bed sore, as the skin is damaged by continual pressure on it. With motor neurone disease, you will be unlikely to want to stay in one position for long and will need to have your position changed regularly. As a result, bed sores are rare in people with motor neurone disease. Your occupational therapist can advise you on the use of special cushions in your wheelchair, to help you be more comfortable. If a sore should develop, your nurse will be able to advise on the most suitable treatment.

Why do I keep crying?

Occasionally some people find that, for no obvious reason, they burst into tears or else start to cry or laugh over a small incident that would never have affected them before. This can be very frightening as it feels as if the emotions are out of control. This symptom occurs as part of the disease of MND, and is probably related to changes within the frontal lobe – the front part of the brain. Research has shown that this area may become involved in MND and the control of the emotions may be affected. So what would normally have led to a smile can cause an outburst of laughing, and a sad incident can lead to bursting into tears, instead of just a feeling of sadness. If the cause of these emotional outbursts is understood, it may be easier to cope with them. It is also possible to explain the reason for the tears to your family and friends, who may otherwise be bewildered by these changes.

Feelings of depression and anxiety are only to be expected when someone has been diagnosed with a serious disease – these feelings are part of a normal reaction to this news. It is important to share these concerns with others, particularly with your family, as they may be experiencing similar feelings and need the opportunity to talk as well. If these feelings come to dominate your life or continue for longer, though, discuss your concerns with your doctor or nurse. Talking with them may be all you need, but if you need more help, a counsellor or social worker may allow these feelings to be shared. Sometimes medication may be needed to help you overcome these problems, such as diazepam for anxiety, or antidepressants, such as amitriptyline, sertraline or fluoxetine, if you have become depressed. If you need extra help in the form of medication, this is not a sign of weakness. The drugs will merely help you to cope with the illness and the problems it causes.

Although at the moment there is no treatment available that can cure motor neurone disease, there are many ways in which the effects of the disease can be overcome or lessened. Every person is different and the cause of each problem must be found so that any treatment can be as effective as possible, but there is help for the problems associated with the disease. The various options available will enable you to live life as fully as possible.

5

How will my family cope?

Introduction

Most people are part of a family, and the shock and anxiety felt by you will be shared by those close to you. Your family members may have questions and concerns that they would like to discuss but, all too often, people avoid such discussion as they are afraid of upsetting the others. It is understandable that no one wants to upset those close to them, but *not* sharing these concerns may, in fact, lead to more problems.

The aim of this chapter is to enable you and your family to ask questions and talk about the effects of the condition on everyone, for how you feel will affect those close to you and their feelings will, in turn, affect you.

How can I talk about motor neurone disease with my family?

During the changes that have occurred before the diagnosis of motor neurone disease has been made, your family will have been concerned about your condition, and you may all have wondered what was happening to you. You may find it helpful to see the doctors and nurses with a family member so that you both can hear the details of how the various tests are carried out and, later, the results of these tests. That way, you and your family can share the experience and learn about the condition together. However, if this is not possible, you may want to ask for a chance to see the doctor again with your family so that they can be more closely involved.

After hearing the diagnosis of motor neurone disease, you may all feel shocked and frightened. All of you may be unsure about how it will affect you, and you may have read or heard accounts in the newspapers and other media that highlight the distressing effects of the disease. It may be helpful to talk about the disease and read more about it (such as the information given in Chapter 1). This may not be easy and may be upsetting, but this distress is very natural and sharing it can only help you and your family cope with the problems you may encounter as the condition develops.

How do we cope with what is happening?

As you saw in Chapters 2 and 4, there are many changes that can occur as motor neurone disease progresses. The combination of changes experienced will vary from person to person, as everyone is affected differently. Thus, you and your family will face different problems from those faced by anyone else, although many will have faced and coped with *similar* situations.

Your family need to be included in the care you may need and the plans that need to be made. It is important to share how the problems are affecting you and to explain how you would like to be helped. On occasion, other people may try to help *too* much and, inadvertently, stop you doing what you want to do, but at times they may not realize what your needs are and leave you feeling frustrated. The only way to overcome these difficulties is to talk about your own problems and feelings and listen to those of your family. In this way, you can all share in the process of working out the best way of coping for all of you. If these problems are not shared, there may be conflict between you and your family, and all of you are likely to become increasingly frustrated and angry.

Often families just try to carry on as normally as possible, trying to ignore the effects of the disease. Although the aim in caring for someone with motor neurone disease *is* to keep life as normal as possible, it is *also* important to face the changes that are occurring head on. The disease will not go away if it is ignored, and the time will come when it will be necessary to make changes to some of the normal activities of the household. At first these changes may be small, but as you become weaker, the changes from the normal routine will need to be greater. Everyone needs to accept that these changes have to occur, and they should be discussed.

What about my children?

Children are part of many families and need to be included in the discussions and plans that you are all considering, regardless of their age. Obviously how well children understand the disease will vary and will depend on their age, but even the youngest children will realize that all is not well and sense the worries and feelings of unease that their parents and grandparents are experiencing. Many families try to keep the children out of any discussions, not wanting to worry them, but this may, in fact, *increase* children's fears as they may feel rejected and be afraid that, in some way, they may be to blame for the disease. In turn, children may not want to worry *you*, and will need to be asked about their worries and concerns. You may become aware from their questions that they are unsettled or, on occasions, their schoolwork may worsen. It is important to let the teachers know the situation at home so that the children can be handled sensitively if there are any changes in behaviour. Also, a teacher may be able to talk more easily with the children about their worries and, if the teacher knows what is happening, he or she can answer any questions truthfully.

Children may be frightened by some of the changes that are happening to you as the condition worsens. The muscle weakness and speech problems may seem very strange to a child, as even adults find this difficult. Children may also be embarrassed by the changes and try to avoid being seen with a person who is obviously 'different' and 'ill'.

A social worker or counsellor may also be able to help you to talk with your child or children, and will be able to discuss with you possible ways of helping them to talk about their worries. Equally, some children find it easier to talk to people outside the family as there is no fear of upsetting them, so it can be worth their having some sessions alone with a social worker or counsellor. Some children may also find it easier to express their concerns in the form of pictures or stories rather than talking about them.

The Motor Neurone Disease Association has produced a small workbook for young children entitled *When Someone Close Has MND*. This explains a little about the disease in simple terms and provides an opportunity for the child to discuss its contents with you or another adult. Remember, too, that often children can cope with difficult news much better than we, as parents, expect them to. They do need an opportunity to talk, though, and have some of their questions answered in a simple way so that they can understand what is happening and what may happen in the future. It is important to be truthful and open – if children find out later that someone has lied to them, they will lose confidence in that person and may never be able to trust him or her again.

Children in their teenage years may find it particularly difficult to talk about their worries, but they find the disease even more of a threat to them. During the teenage years, there are many mixed feelings about parents. Teenagers are trying to make sense of the changes occurring in themselves and the changing relationships with their parents and friends. It is helpful to give them time to talk about these worries. Again, their worries may come out as problems at school, so their teachers need to be aware of what is happening. The help a teacher or social worker can give may be particularly beneficial.

How can I help my family?

When facing the challenges of motor neurone disease, you will need a lot of support and your family will be very important in providing this help. They will *also* need support and you will, in turn, be able to help *them*. To enable you all to cope with the changes the disease brings, you will need to be able to share your feelings, concerns and fears. You need to be able to talk and discuss your own worries and listen to their concerns. This will only happen if you are all open and truthful with each other, and one of the most important ways in which you can help your family is to allow this to happen.

You will need to be able to share your feelings with those close to you, not hide them. Any attempt to hide your emotions will often fail – your family will usually see through the front you put up. Equally, you will probably realize when they are trying to hide things from you. If some feelings *are* hidden, they may make the worries worse – your family may suspect that there is something wrong but will not know what the problem is. They may then feel unable to talk about their own worries because they may fear that this will just make it worse. Thus, it all becomes more of a problem than is necessary. Openness and sharing will help to stop such misunderstandings occurring and allow you and your family to cope with the progress of the disease.

What about sex?

Your sexual needs may be a very important part of your relationship and should not be ignored. Motor neurone disease does not affect sexual ability or the ability to have an erection, and an orgasm will remain unchanged.

Despite illness or age, we all have a need to express our sexuality and to show our feelings towards those we love. There are many ways in which these feelings may be expressed, and all couples are different, having their own particular ways of expressing their love for each other. When one partner becomes disabled, the relationship will change and it may no longer be possible to express yourself in the ways you are used to. This can be confusing and difficult for both partners in the relationship, and these concerns need to be discussed. Some people may find it difficult to talk about these changes, but if they are ignored, resentment may develop.

Many of us find it difficult to discuss our sexual needs and preferences, even with our partners. The changes that result from the disease, such as difficulties in moving or the discomfort felt in certain positions, may change sex from an enriching experience to a time of fear and pain. Only by talking about these changes and looking at alternative positions and so on will you be able to improve the situation. For example, if you are a man and find movement difficult, try having sex with your partner on top or vice versa if you are a woman. In this way, instead of being a time of distress, this can be a time of experimentation and enjoyment.

If sex ultimately becomes too difficult in any position, consider other ways of showing your affection and allowing your sexuality to be expressed, such as stimulation by masturbation or oral sex.

Sex itself may become less of an issue for some couples, but do make sure that you continue to show your love in other ways. Even if you do not want sex, you can still cuddle and kiss! A person with motor neurone disease has to cope with so many changes, but you still need to be able to show your affection for your partner and those close to you, and receive it from them. Some members of the family may need permission to show that they care, but encourage them to behave normally. If they would normally give you a hug and a kiss, they should still feel able to do so now that you have the disease. If, say, hugs cause discomfort, tell them and work out an alternative.

Will my family be affected too?

As discussed in Chapter 1, the disease can run in a family for a small number of people and there could then be an increased risk to your children. However, these forms of the disease – known as familial MND – are rarer and affect only 5–10 per cent of all people with the disease.

If you do think that someone in your family has been affected by the disease in the past, talk to your neurologist so that the risks can be assessed.

There are now three genes known that may be abnormal and lead to MND:

- The superoxide dismutase (SOD1) gene – the abnormal gene appears to produce an abnormal protein that damages the cell. This accounts for about 20 per cent of all familial cases of MND, that is 1 per cent of all people with MND.
- TDP-43 – changes in this gene cause the production of abnormal protein in the cell, which is thought to harm the cell. This seems to account for 3–5 per cent of people with familial MND, although as the abnormal TDP-43 protein has been found in people with no family history, it may be involved in all people with the disease. This is still being investigated.
- FUS (fused in sarcoma) – this gene is involved in how cells make proteins, but the exact mechanism is not known. This accounts for about 3–5 per cent of all people with familial MND.

It is now possible to test for changes in the SOD1 gene, and it may be possible in the future to test for the other abnormal genes. However, any testing should be considered only after careful discussion and thought, and your neurologist and specialist genetic counselling teams should be involved. It is difficult to decide if you would wish family members to be tested, as a positive result would show that there is a very greatly increased likelihood of developing motor neurone disease, even if the person shows no sign of the disease at the present time. Knowing that the disease may develop later in their life might be too much for many people. The knowledge may be important to some who, knowing the risks and the possibility of passing on the abnormal gene to their children, may decide against having children at all.

For the vast majority of people with motor neurone disease, there is *no* known risk of passing on the disease to their children, either by an infection or in their genes. It may be helpful to discuss your concerns and worries about these issues within the family, however, as some people may be fearful and even avoid visiting for fear of catching the disease.

How can we manage the family finances?

There may be many financial problems to cope with as a family as a result of having motor neurone disease. If you are unable to continue working full-time, it may be necessary to consider part-time working, having time off or taking early retirement. If you require extra help at home, your partner may also have to change their work and so the financial losses may be increased as a result. These changes may greatly affect a family, especially if there are children, who may find it difficult to appreciate why there have to be changes in the family budget and possible restrictions on spending.

There are several allowances and benefits that can be obtained, and these are described more fully in Chapter 9. Some people find it difficult to apply for these, as they do not want to ask for 'charity'. However, as a taxpayer, you have contributed towards these allowances when working and so you are entitled to claim them if you are unable to continue working because of your illness.

It may be necessary to discuss with your employer or the personnel department the possibility of early retirement. The exact benefits received will vary from individual to individual, and careful assessment of your particular situation will be necessary. A social worker or benefits adviser may be able to give you advice as to which is the best option, or a Citizens' Advice Bureau or some other advice centres could offer useful independent advice. The decisions that need to be made for you and your family may be difficult, and such advice can help you and your family work out what options are the best for you all.

What help can we get?

Any illness brings about all sorts of difficulties as the normal patterns of life are disrupted. Motor neurone disease affects so many aspects of daily living – from the most basic hurdle of coping with becoming a disabled person, to the financial questions that have to be answered when work is no longer possible, particularly if a family member also gives up work to help you.

It may be necessary to ask for extra help, either of a practical nature, such as with household chores or nursing, or with finances. It is important to be willing to ask and accept help *before* a crisis develops. It may be more difficult to arrange the necessary help in a hurry, when everything has gone wrong and a crisis has developed. Such a crisis can be prevented if a little extra help is provided in time.

If you need help with things of a personal nature, such as bathing or help with the toilet, talk to your GP and community nurse. Your community nurse can then assess the situation and help you all make the necessary plans to cope with it. The local social services department may also be able to provide help, and a care manager or social worker can come and discuss with you and your family what they could do for you (see also page 66). There may be charges for this help, though.

The financial implications that follow from being ill, such as not being able to work or being made redundant or maybe needing to retire early on grounds of ill health, can be worrying. A social worker or care manager can provide advice on the various allowances that can be claimed (see Chapter 9 for more details). There are often delays, and so it is important to find out what can be claimed and fill in the necessary forms before there is a financial crisis. Discuss your position with the personnel department at your place of employment as it may be to your advantage to consider early retirement.

There are many other organizations that may be able to help you and your family – for example the Motor Neurone Disease Association (see Chapter 8), Crossroads Care, Age UK and the British Red Cross (these are described under their entries in the Useful addresses section).

If it becomes difficult to talk with your family about the disease and how it is affecting you, you may need to discuss this with someone. If there is a counsellor or social worker at the neurology centre, they may be able to help. Your own GP or community nurse may also be able to help you talk together or refer you to a counsellor who can help. The Motor Neurone Disease Association's regional care development adviser for your area may also be able to answer your questions and help you as a family to talk more easily together about how to make the best of what is available.

It may also be helpful to meet other people who have the disease. The Motor Neurone Disease Association's local branches meet regularly and offer the chance to do just this, sharing experiences and advice. However, it must always be remembered that everyone's experience of the disease is different, so that the advice you get from someone else may not always apply or be helpful to you.

6

Facing the future

Introduction

As the disease progresses, there are more and more changes to be faced. The changes that you may have to cope with may be different from those experienced by other people with motor neurone disease because the disease affects different people in different ways. However, everyone has to face increasing disability as the disease progresses. These changes will affect your family and all of you may have concerns and fears for the future that need to be shared.

What will happen as I become more ill?

As the disease progresses, all the symptoms and difficulties outlined in Chapter 4 become more likely to occur. There is no definite pattern to the changes and every person is different. However, certain changes are common to everyone who has the disease – in strength, breathing, swallowing and speech.

Will I become weaker?

As more nerves become affected by the disease, your muscles will become weaker. Depending on which cells are affected (see pages 3–4), the muscles may feel very weak and floppy or weak and stiff. The effects of the weakness will depend on the muscles involved. Quite often, the neck muscles become weaker and, as a result, the head tends to fall forwards and the chin rests on the chest. This can be both uncomfortable and inconvenient as you may not be able to see ahead easily. Your physiotherapist can advise you on the possible use of a collar or neck support to help you.

As the legs become weaker, walking may become more difficult. It may become necessary to consider using an aid of some sort to help with walking, especially if your balance is affected. Using a walking stick or frame or a wheelchair may be helpful (see page 29).

If the muscles of the arms are affected by the disease, it may be necessary to have extra help with moving into and out of a chair or moving in bed. An electrically operated chair can help move you from sitting to standing and so help you remain more independent.

There are also bed elevators that allow you to control the angle of the bed and sit up in bed using a hand switch. If movement in bed becomes more difficult, there are specially designed beds that help your carers move you more easily. Your occupational therapist will be able to advise you on what is available and how to use this equipment.

Other muscles may become weaker, including the muscles of your abdomen. If these become very weak it may be difficult to push when you need to go to the toilet. There are ways to get over this problem (see page 32).

Will my breathing worsen?

If the muscles that you use in breathing are affected by the disease, breathing may become more difficult and you may feel breathless when you are mobile or even while resting (see page 23). Medication (such as diazepam or morphine) is often very helpful in reducing the feelings of breathlessness. Many people, including doctors and nurses, worry about the use of morphine as they fear that it may well shorten life. However, if morphine is used carefully, it can reduce distress, such as pain and breathlessness, with few side-effects and without causing harm.

If there is a *sudden* change in your breathing, or coughing and spluttering occurs, it may be necessary to have an injection so that the problem is relieved as quickly as possible. The injection is usually of a painkiller (such as morphine), a relaxing drug (such as midazolam) and a drug to reduce the secretions in the lung and relax the muscles of the airways (such as hyoscine). Such an injection acts within a few minutes and quickly controls the breathing. It will usually make you feel drowsy. Many people are concerned when injections are given as they may fear an injection could shorten life, but this combination of drugs is effective in helping to relieve the problem and does not necessarily hasten death (see also page 79 regarding the Just in Case kit).

Weakness of the breathing muscles may lead to problems, as the body is not able to get sufficient oxygen or is not able to clear the waste carbon dioxide from the body – this is known as respiratory failure. These problems may occur particularly at night, as the breathing muscles work less effectively when you lie down. A person with these problems may wake during the night, feel more breathless when lying down, have bad dreams or nightmares, have a headache or feel hung-over in the morning, feel tired, have difficulty concentrating and remembering things, have a poorer appetite and be muddled during the day.

If you have these problems, do discuss them with your doctors and nurses. They may check your breathing on a regular basis, at your appointments, using special testing machines, and may also check the oxygen level in your blood using a finger probe (a pulse oximeter). If it is found that there are abnormalities, further tests would be made.

There is evidence that a machine to help the breathing may be helpful if someone has these problems. This is called non-invasive ventilation (NIV). A mask is fitted on the face and a ventilator helps to support the breathing by pushing air into the lungs. This can be particularly helpful if there are problems at night, and the use of NIV may help you feel better in the morning and throughout the day. There is also evidence from research that this may extend life.

However, not everyone can cope with the mask and ventilator when using NIV. If someone has swallowing problems and tends to dribble, the mask may not be helpful, and some people find it is too claustrophobic. It is important to discuss the issues with your doctors and nurses so that everyone is clear as to your wishes. The NIV will help your symptoms but it does not affect the disease itself and so the body will continue to weaken. Some people find this too difficult and may ask to stop the ventilation (see page 50).

On occasions, consideration may be given to using a ventilator to take over breathing all the time. This is a more serious step as a tracheostomy has to be made. Under anaesthetic, a small cut is made in the neck so that a tube can be put into the windpipe below the voice box. A ventilator can then be attached to the tube and the machine does the breathing for you.

This obviously has a great effect on your life as you then need continuous nursing care because you can never be left alone in case the ventilator goes wrong. Also, speech is very difficult and you are restricted in the range of activities you can do; the machine always has to go with you although there are small, portable ventilators available that can be attached to a wheelchair.

Despite the help with breathing a ventilator can give you, the disease can continue to worsen until you become totally dependent on others. Thus deciding whether or not to use a ventilator is very difficult as there are so many aspects of this care to be considered by you and your family. In addition, in the UK at the time of writing, there are not enough resources to offer this help to many people. Often this form of treatment is used only if the disease has been diagnosed after the breathing problems and the use of the ventilator has started.

As there are many difficulties associated with using a ventilator, this form of treatment should only be considered after much discussion of all the aspects as they affect you and those close to you. Remember, too, that once a ventilator is used it may be difficult to stop using it later as you will then be unable to breathe alone.

Will my problems with swallowing get worse?

Not everyone with motor neurone disease will develop problems with swallowing, but for some it will become an increasing problem, and alternative ways of feeding yourself may need to be considered. A percutaneous endoscopic gastrostomy (PEG) may be helpful for some people, when eating has become an ordeal.

A PEG is inserted in hospital and requires only a short stay – usually only a day or two. You are given an injection to make you feel sleepy, but not a general anaesthetic. The doctor then passes an endoscope (a special, fine fibre-optic cable flexible telescope) into your mouth and down into the stomach. A small area of skin on your tummy is injected with a local anaesthetic and a little cut made in the skin. A needle is then pushed into the stomach and a wire passed through and pulled up to your mouth as the endoscope is pulled upwards. A tube is then passed over this wire and then the wire and tube are pulled back down into your stomach and out of the small cut in the abdominal wall. The tube is then fixed in place using a special plastic fixator, and a stitch may be made to ensure that the tube does not become loose.

The whole operation only takes 15 to 30 minutes and you wake fully a few hours later. The insertion of a PEG should not be painful, although you may feel some discomfort when the endoscope is passed down into the stomach.

Once a PEG has been inserted, it will be tested by putting some water down the tube. Feeding via the tube can start soon after the tube is inserted, and a dietitian will be able to advise on the feeds that can be used. During feeding, the tube is connected to a pump that slowly pushes the liquid food through the tube and into the stomach. The timing of feeds can be decided by you, taking into account the advice of a dietitian.

Once the cut has completely healed, you can have a bath, and even swim, as long as the tube is closed off. When the tube is not being used for feeding, it can be kept taped to the stomach and is hardly noticeable.

The decision as to whether or not to have a PEG inserted can be a very difficult one. The fact that you need to consider using an artificial method of feeding can be hard to accept, and there are often fears that having the tube there will restrict what you can do. However, a PEG will allow you to feed your body without the problems that may have been experienced, such as long and distressing meals. Certain foods can still be taken normally and, in the first few weeks after it has been inserted, the majority of food may be taken normally and the PEG used only to top up these meals to ensure that you do not become malnourished. Some people may not even use their PEG at first, keeping it in reserve in case feeding becomes more troublesome. If your breathing has become difficult, it may be necessary to discuss in more depth the insertion of a PEG: there are increased risks if the insertion is delayed for too long because your breathing could become worse during the procedure.

Anyone whose ability to swallow worsens should consider having a PEG inserted. It is important to discuss the whole issue with your carers, nurses, doctors, dietitian or any other professional, and it may be helpful to discuss the pros and cons of a PEG with others too, particularly with someone who has a PEG themselves.

An alternative feeding tube may be used on occasion. This is called an RIG – radiologically inserted gastrostomy – or PRG – percutaneous radiological gastrostomy. This tube can be inserted more easily and without the need to give any medication to make you sleepy. What happens is that a small tube is passed through the nose into the stomach and then some dye is given through the tube, so that the doctor can see the stomach. After the skin is made numb with a local anaesthetic, the RIG tube is inserted and secured with some stitches. This tube can be inserted if there is evidence of breathing problems, and if necessary, the non-invasive ventilation (NIV) system can be continued throughout the procedure. The stitches are removed after a few days and the tube can be used immediately, in exactly the same way as a PEG. The procedure is safer for someone with breathing difficulties, and its use may be considered on occasion.

What else may happen?

As everyone is so different, it is impossible to know how motor neurone disease will affect you. The various possibilities are described in Chapter 4, and as the disease progresses, any of these problems may occur, but how they will affect you cannot be predicted. It is important to share with your family and your doctor, nurse and other carers how you are feeling and any changes that you notice. It is then possible for problems to be fully assessed and appropriate action taken, whether this means the prescription of medication or advice being given on how to cope with this new symptom. All along, there needs to be cooperation, and all those involved in helping you need to work together so that you are able to stay as independent as possible and carry on as normally as possible, despite the disease.

Will I become confused?

As someone facing a disease that worsens over time, you may be worried about whether your brain will be affected and your thinking altered. In the past it was thought that only a small proportion of people with MND were affected in this way, but recent research has shown that there may be cognitive change – this may affect the way a person thinks through activities, concentrates, carries out tasks, communicates, and interacts with and responds to other people.

The research has shown that people with MND may be in one of four groups:

- people with no cognitive change
- people with subtle cognitive or behavioural changes
- people with severe changes, known as frontotemporal dementia
- people with frontotemporal dementia who later develop MND.

Dementia may be present in about 5–15 per cent of people with MND, but the subtle changes may occur in many more people – although they may not always be recognized. These subtle changes include difficulties in concentration, planning activities, making decisions, holding a conversation or doing activities (which may be difficult if there are distractions), finishing activities, remembering names of items that would have been known before, feeling restless, eating foods when not necessarily hungry, acting impulsively, becoming fixated on one routine or activity or seeming to be indifferent to the distress or feelings of someone close. All this may be difficult for both you and your family.

If you do feel that you may have problems, do discuss them with your family and the doctors and nurses. If they know that you find some activities difficult, they can make arrangements to make them easier for you and will be able to understand why you are behaving as you are. It may also be important to consider advance care planning while you are able to make important decisions – see pages 56–8.

Will I become incontinent?

Motor neurone disease will not affect the nerves that control the bladder (see page 4) and so you will not normally lose control and become incontinent. However, you may have trouble going to the toilet because of some other problem, such as a urine infection or, in the case of men, an enlarged prostate gland. If you have difficulty walking, getting to a toilet in time might be difficult. All these kinds of problems can usually be overcome – an infection can be treated with antibiotics and, with forward planning and care, you can ensure that you reach the toilet in plenty of time. It may not *always* be possible to treat the cause of the problem though, and on occasions, it may be necessary to consider the use of a catheter. A catheter is a tube that is passed into the bladder through the urethra (where the urine leaves the body). There is only a little discomfort when this is done and it passes within a few minutes.

How will I die?

For many of us there is a greater fear of the *process* of dying than of death itself. With motor neurone disease such fears may be greater as there is often a fear of choking and breathlessness. Unfortunately, much has been written about people choking to death, both in the newspapers and in other articles about motor neurone disease. If care has been taken to reduce your various symptoms as the disease has progressed, choking and breathlessness are rare and, for most people, there is no such dramatic event at the time of death but, rather, a peaceful ending.

Most of us have our own particular fears about our future and death. All of us have our own experiences and memories of other family members and friends who have died. For some, it will be the unknown that is frightening, as you may never have been involved in the care of someone as death approaches. Your fears of the unknown will affect you in many different ways, and you will usually find it helpful to talk about them and your other feelings about dying as openly as possible with both your family and the professionals involved in your care. In this way, many of your fears can be reduced.

Usually there is a gradual weakening and increasing sleepiness. Breathing may become weaker, but with the correct medication, this is not distressing. Consciousness reduces as the body becomes weaker, and the moment of death comes peacefully as the breathing slowly reduces, both in depth and frequency and, finally, ceases. On occasion, the breathing may change shortly before death, with the depth of the breaths varying over the course of a few minutes from deeper breaths to much shallower ones and, for a few moments, the breathing may stop altogether and then restart. This kind of breathing is known as Cheyne-Stokes respiration, and it occurs shortly before death.

What can be done if I should choke?

Choking is very rare as a cause of death if there has been the opportunity adequately to treat the problems associated with breathing and swallowing earlier in the course of the disease. It is important that swallowing does not become so difficult that saliva dribbles from the mouth or goes back into the throat and causes coughing and spluttering. As we have seen, the amount of saliva produced can be reduced by taking appropriate medication (see page 25), and the insertion of a PEG (see page 50) may be helpful if swallowing becomes very difficult. Feelings of breathlessness can also be eased by the careful use of medication (see page 79).

If these problems have been monitored and treated, the chances of increased breathlessness and choking occurring are further reduced. However, many people still fear that they might choke. The Motor Neurone Disease Association has developed the Just in Case kit to help allay these fears. The kit allows medication to be available in the house at all times so that it can be used to control a choking attack if one should occur. The kit includes a box for the medication and a booklet that gives instructions on the most suitable medication to use. The booklet can be discussed by you and your family with your GP and the community nurse. If everyone agrees that the kit will be helpful, your GP can prescribe the medication, which is then stored in the box, together with the booklet. If a choking attack should occur, any doctor or nurse – even if not your usual carers – will be able to read the instructions and give you the medication without any delay. It may also be possible, if you and your family feel comfortable with the idea, for medication to be given while waiting for the doctor or nurse to come. The medication, midazolam, can be given in the mouth, and is absorbed quickly from the gums, without the need to swallow anything or have an injection. It can be administered with a small syringe by a family member or carer, and will help the person to relax and relieve any distress until outside help arrives.

For most people, the Just in Case kit will never be needed, but like an insurance policy, it is there if it is required. It does ensure that all the necessary medication is quickly available and that its use has been discussed by you, your family and doctor and nurse. If your breathing or ability to swallow are becoming more difficult or if you are concerned that a choking attack may occur, it may be helpful to consider having the kit, so that you are all prepared if the worst should occur.

What else can I do?

From 2005 the Mental Capacity Act has provided a legal framework for people to say what they would wish to happen for their care if they were unable to tell their carers at the time. This may be of help to people with MND, especially as we now know that the brain may be affected and in particular that decision-making may be difficult for some people.

Individuals can make arrangements for their care in the event that they are no longer able to make the decisions for themselves. If you are able to make decisions clearly yourself, the doctors and nurses will always ask you about your wishes. However, if you are unable to make the decisions, because you are confused or unconscious, the doctor will have to make the decisions for you in 'your best interests', using any information available about your wishes, and involving your family, as appropriate. You may express your wishes in different ways:

- An advance statement – this is a statement about your wishes, but it may not be specific to MND and is not legally binding. However, a doctor should take it into consideration when making decisions on your behalf.
- An advance decision to refuse treatment – you can complete a specific form expressing your wishes about treatments you would not wish to receive (such as tracheostomy, cardio-pulmonary resuscitation (restarting your heart), admission to hospital), providing that it is stated that you realize that this may put your life at risk and it is specific for these circumstances of MND. This document, if completed correctly and witnessed, is legally binding, and everyone should take note of it when treating you.
- A lasting power of attorney – you may complete forms stating whom you would like to make decisions on your behalf if you are unable to make these decisions yourself. There are two forms – one for your personal welfare (health and social care decisions) – and one for your property and affairs (financial decisions). You may define anyone to take on these roles and complete the forms and have them registered at the Office of the Public Guardian. If you are unable to make decisions, the

person with your power of attorney would be able to do so on your behalf.

These issues may be difficult for you to discuss with your doctors and nurses and family, but by making your wishes known it may be a great help to them and reassuring for you. There are other ways in which you can make your wishes known, and this is known as advance care planning. You may wish to state your preferred place of care or death and other aspects of care.

How can I take my medicines?

If it becomes more difficult to swallow, it may be impossible for you to take any tablets or even liquid medicines. It is usually necessary to continue with the medication, though, because as you become less well, it is more important to make sure that your symptoms are controlled as well as possible. There are several ways in which you can ensure that the medication is still given. It can be given in liquid form, through a tube, such as a PEG or PRG (see pages 50–2), suppositories, injections or an injection system (see below).

Many of the medications used to control the symptoms of motor neurone disease are available in a liquid form. Some people find that they are able to take their medication in liquid form when taking tablets becomes difficult, but others find that swallowing liquids is even more troublesome, and then other methods must be used.

There are some medicines that are available in the form of suppositories. The medication can then be given by inserting the suppository into the rectum, avoiding the need to swallow. Some people find this form of medication very helpful, but others do not like the idea of using suppositories. However, they may be preferable to having injections. If you have haemorrhoids (piles) or you are very constipated or have diarrhoea, then you will not be able to use suppositories.

Another way of taking medication is via injections. On occasion it may only be necessary to have one or two injections to
settle a problem, such as severe dribbling or sickness, and then
the medication might be able to be continued by mouth. If,
however, you will need to continue to have your medication
injected, an injection system may be used. A small needle is
placed under the skin and covered with a transparent dressing.
The tubing from this needle is connected up to a syringe of the
medication that you need and the syringe is fitted to a small
machine, called a syringe driver or syringe pump. This slowly
pushes the plunger of the syringe so that the medication enters
your system slowly over the next 24 hours. Your nurse can then
change the syringe each day, and where the needle is inserted
is not painful. The syringe driver is small and can be carried in
a shoulder holster or a pouch so that it does not restrict you in
your day-to-day activities. Using a syringe driver allows medication to be given without needing to swallow, and makes sure
that the symptoms are controlled as well as possible. The needle
is repositioned every few days and your medication can be given
in this way for as long as is necessary.

Where can I be cared for?

As you become less well it may be necessary to consider, with
your family, how and where you will be cared for. Most people
prefer to be at home with their families, but much consideration
and planning may be necessary for this to be possible. Extra
help may be necessary, ranging from nursing help to help with
personal issues such as going to the toilet and bathing or with
the household chores and shopping. If possible, these plans
should be made *before* a crisis is reached. Your doctor, nurse,
care manager or social worker, physiotherapist or occupational
therapist may be able to help you and your family in making
these decisions (see Chapter 7, where their roles are discussed).

Extra equipment, to help with moving or with going to the toilet, may be needed, as well as the extra practical help.

With careful planning and preparation, many people are able to stay at home. There is often a great strain on everyone involved, and sometimes a period of rest allows the care at home to continue. For instance, attending a day centre or a day hospice allows your family a break for at least part of one day, so that they can get some jobs done or have time to themselves, knowing that you are being cared for. Sometimes, admission to a hospital, neurological centre or a hospice for a period of one to two weeks allows a family a break from caring and also enables hospital or hospice staff closely to supervise and reassess your symptoms.

If you do not have close family who are able to care for you at home, you may still be able to stay at home alone, even as you become less well and more disabled. Much planning and help may be needed to do this, however, and it may not always be available. It may then be necessary to look at being cared for in a hospice or nursing home. Most hospices are able to offer admission to people with motor neurone disease. Many worry that a hospice is a gloomy or dismal place, but the reality is often very different. The aim of the caring team in a hospice is to help you to be independent and active and to maintain control over your life for as long as possible. However, many hospices are only able to offer a short period of care, of a few weeks. If longer-term care is needed, it may be necessary to think about a nursing home.

Many nursing homes are able to take disabled people, and not all the residents are necessarily elderly. A nurse is always present in a nursing home and will be able to help you if there is a crisis. It would be necessary to discuss this option with both your family and your care manager or social worker from social services (see page 66) as plans may need to be made and the financial arrangements clarified. There is a charge for nursing home care, but the local social services department will meet all or a proportion of the costs if your savings and income are below certain levels.

Making these decisions is not easy, but they do need to be made.

It is best to prepare ahead rather than have to decide in a crisis, such as when your carers find that they are no longer able to cope or become ill themselves. Sometimes hospices or nursing home care will never be needed, but at least the preparations will have been made and be known to everyone involved in your care should the need arise.

7

Who will be caring for me?

Introduction

Many people will be involved in your care, both in hospital and at home. This chapter tries to explain the roles of the professionals, and other agencies, with whom you may come into contact.

Neurologist

A neurologist is a hospital specialist who sees people who have, or are thought to have, diseases of the nervous system. The neurologist will usually be based in a hospital, often at a neurological centre, although, increasingly, some specialists do see people at the GP's surgery. A neurologist aims to find the cause of your symptoms and suggests treatment, if this is possible.

Often, the tests and investigations needed will have to be carried out in hospital over the course of a few days, and you will need to stay in hospital while they are done. This may take place in your local hospital, but often you will have to go to a larger neurological centre, which may be away from your own town or city. The neurological centre has more facilities for carrying out tests on the nervous system than do most local hospitals – there will be more specialized equipment there, and doctors and nurses who specialize in the care of people with diseases of the nervous system.

While in hospital, you may meet several doctors:

- **a consultant** – the specialist, the most senior doctor in charge of your care

- **a specialist registrar** – a doctor who is training to be a specialist
- **a senior house officer** – a more junior doctor, whom you may see regularly
- **a house officer** – a newly qualified doctor who is responsible for your day-to-day care.

If you have questions, you should always feel able to ask them of any of the doctors so that you can be clear as to what is involved in the various tests and discuss the results with them afterwards.

Consultant in rehabilitation medicine

After you have been diagnosed, you may be referred to a consultant in rehabilitation medicine. This is a specialist involved in the assessment and care of people with disabilities. They may be able to advise you on the best way to maintain your mobility and independence, including the provision of walking aids, appliances, wheelchairs and environmental control systems. They are usually based at disablement service centres. Although you may be seen more locally at first, it may be necessary to go to a centre (which again may be away from your home town) for a full assessment and to have the opportunity to try the various aids. Each centre has skilled therapists and rehabilitation engineers who will be able to advise you as to the best aid or aids for your particular needs.

Hospital nurses

While in hospital, you will be cared for by a team of nurses. On most wards, you will be told who your named nurse is, and that nurse will be primarily responsible for your care while you are a patient on that ward. When your named nurse is not on duty, another member of the nursing team will take over responsibility for your care. If you have any questions or worries, do ask your nurse. If your nurse is not able to provide an answer, he or she should be able to ask the doctors or another member of the team for advice.

There are different grades of nurses:

- **ward sister** or **manager,** who runs the ward
- **staff nurse** – a fully qualified nurse
- **healthcare assistant**, who will care for you under the supervision of a staff nurse.

In some hospitals, there may also be clinical nurse specialists who give the specialized support required by some patients. There may be a nurse specialist in a neurological centre who helps with the care of patients with serious illnesses, such as motor neurone disease, and liaises with all the other professional carers and you and your family, to make sure that your care is coordinated to avoid duplication or omissions and that everyone knows what is planned. The nurse specialist will also be able to spend time with you and your family, to explain the disease to you, and support you at this time.

GP

Your GP will usually be well known to you as you will have needed to have seen him or her before for other illnesses and so on. The GP will probably be the first doctor you will see when you first develop symptoms and he or she will refer you to the other specialists.

For a GP, motor neurone disease will be a rare condition – typically GPs see only one or two people with the disease in their career. The Motor Neurone Disease Association produces a very informative pack of leaflets for doctors, nurses and other professional carers, and you should encourage your GP to obtain these from the Association's national office or your regional care development adviser. The Royal College of General Practitioners has also produced a booklet on motor neurone disease, and your GP may find this useful too.

Your GP will be the main doctor involved in your care at home and will help to ensure that all the services you need are available to you. If you feel that you need to ask questions, GPs are there to provide answers, and if they do not immediately know, they should be able to find out the information that you need. If you find it difficult to get out of the house and to the surgery, your GP will visit you at home. Your GP will have a very important part to play in your care at home, and you will both need to help each other and work together as a partnership.

Community nurse

While you are at home, the local community nurse (or district nurse) will be able to provide help. The community nurse can help with your nursing and with providing aids, such as bathing aids, mattresses, a hospital-type bed and other helpful devices to use at home. The community nurse will often be part of a wider team and so may come initially to assess your needs. An auxiliary nurse may then come to undertake the nursing care, under the community nurse's supervision. In some areas, there is a twilight nursing service, which can provide a nursing visit in the evening, or a night-nurse visiting service, which is there to provide support at night.

Counsellor or social worker

Many neurological centres may have a counsellor or social worker who is available to help patients and their families.

A counsellor may be able to give you and your family the

opportunity to talk about your fears and concerns at the time you are undergoing the tests, when there may be uncertainty about what is affecting you. A counsellor may also be able to be with you when you see the doctors for the results of the tests, and help you to understand what has been said.

Social workers may also be available in some hospitals. They will also be able to help you and your family cope with the news about the disease. They may also be able to advise you on how to tell your family, especially if there are younger children, and support you all at this time. They are usually a good source of information regarding allowances and benefits that you might be able to claim.

Social services care manager or social worker

Many services can be provided by your local social services department, including practical help at home, occupational therapy assessment, the provision of equipment and alterations to where you live and so on. A care manager or social worker will come to discuss your needs with you and your family and will be able to advise you as to what care can be provided. In some areas this may be restricted, and there will usually be a charge for the service. However, a care manager or social worker may be able to ensure that you get practical help, such as help with getting up, washing, going to the toilet, moving on a regular basis, cooking and shopping and so on. A care manager or social worker may also be able to advise you as to what other services are available in your area.

If you need to consider care in a residential home or nursing home, a care manager or social worker will be able to discuss this with you and, often, can arrange for some or all of this care to be covered, although this will depend on a full assessment of your financial position.

Occupational therapist

An occupational therapist will be able to advise you on what extra help can be provided to allow you to continue to live as normal a life as possible, and will assess your particular needs and work out with you which of your symptoms are causing the most difficulty and what options there are to ameliorate them. An occupational therapist can help you find easier ways to do the many different activities you do every day, including bathing, eating, going to the toilet, moving around and dressing.

Many different aids can be provided that make life more straightforward, such as cutlery with larger handles or a mechanical support for your arm if eating is difficult because your arm tires easily. Advice can be given on the type of clothing you need if your fingers become less nimble or it becomes difficult to dress yourself. There are also aids that can help you bathe yourself, from a simple bath seat, which means that you can stand up again more easily, to a mechanical bathing aid that can lower and raise you in the bath. An occupational therapist will also advise on, and help with the provision of, a wheelchair, should this be necessary. A careful assessment is needed to make sure that the wheelchair is suitable for you and your needs. You may need to have special seating to ensure that you are comfortable, and an electrically powered chair can help you stand up yourself and so remain more independent.

The assessment of your needs will include a look at where you live as it may be necessary to make changes in the house in order for you to remain as independent as possible. Extra rails on the stairs help you climb the stairs more easily and safely. A ramp may be needed at the door so that a wheelchair can go in and out. There may be a need for a lift so that you can go upstairs to bed in your wheelchair. Bigger changes are sometimes necessary, such as converting a downstairs room into a toilet or shower if the stairs become too difficult. Sometimes it may be necessary to extend a room or make other structural changes to allow you to stay in your own home and, rarely, an occupational therapist may need to help you and your family to think about moving if it is not possible to adapt your present home.

Many of these changes may be difficult to accept, as the fact that you have to discuss such aids or changes in your house shows how the disease is affecting you. Often people do not like to talk about this or think about new equipment, and the making of decisions about them is avoided or delayed. This can cause greater problems in the long run, though, as for any large change, such as the installation of a lift, it can take several weeks or even months to obtain and install the aid. Thus, to ensure that a piece of equipment is available for you when it is really needed, it may be necessary to order the equipment some time in advance. Though it is hard, you will need to discuss these issues with your occupational therapist and your family so that you will be prepared as the disease progresses.

Physiotherapist

A physiotherapist will help you to keep as active as possible and maintain maximum movement in the affected muscles. Physiotherapy and exercise are not able to strengthen muscles that have weakened due to motor neurone disease, but they can help to keep them as strong as possible, reduce stiffness, keep the joints flexible and stop the muscles becoming too tight.

Physiotherapy will include exercise, but it may also help you to maintain a good posture and keep stiff muscles moving. A physiotherapist can also advise you if you have problems with your breathing, and show you exercises and techniques to help your breathing.

A physiotherapist will want to include you and your family in the planning of exercises. It is much better for you to undertake the exercises and movements every day, with the help of your family, than to have only one physiotherapy session a week. You will need to take an active part in your physiotherapy plan.

A physiotherapist will be able to help you remain as mobile as possible and use the most suitable walking aid for you, such as a walking stick or frame. A physiotherapist will also advise on other ways of moving and show your family and other carers the best ways to move you if this becomes difficult for you to do on your own. For instance, you may need a hoist to move you from the bed to a chair. It may also be necessary to see what kind of neck support would be best for you if your neck muscles become weaker.

Speech and language therapist

If you have problems with speech or swallowing, a speech and language therapist will be able to assist you, assessing your speech and giving advice on ways of speaking or ensuring that specific aids are provided so that you can continue to communicate as well as possible (see also page 26). He or she may be able to provide communication aids for you to try, or tell you about the nearest communication-aids centre where you can go to try several different systems, before deciding which one best suits you.

A speech and language therapist will also be able to help if you have problems swallowing, examining you as you swallow and giving you advice to improve your swallowing. The therapist may be part of a larger team of experts who will help in this assessment using other tests and examinations.

It is often very helpful to be referred to a speech and language therapist *before* your speech has greatly altered. An early assessment allows the therapist to assess your speech and this can then provide something to measure any later changes against. It also allows the therapist to prepare you and your family for the changes that could possibly occur if the disease progresses and your speech worsens, so you can be aware of what kind of help can be offered.

Dietitian

If swallowing becomes more difficult, a dietitian will be able to advise you on choosing types of food that are easier to swallow, while still maintaining a balanced diet. A dietitian will be able to help you work out the best ways of preparing foods, and will advise on possible supplement foods, such as prepared liquid drinks of milk with added vitamins and minerals, and powdered foods that can be added to your food or drink to make them more nourishing.

If a PEG or PRG (see pages 50–2) becomes necessary, a dietitian will be able to advise you on how this can best help you, will be able to show how the feeds can be given when a PEG is in place and will discuss with you how much food, if any, you will take by this means in the early stages. A dietitian will also monitor your feeding regime and advise on adjusting the amount of food that you take according to how you are feeling or your own particular needs.

Physical disability team

Some areas have a team of professionals specializing in the health and social care of people with physical disabilities. This may be known as a physical disability team, community care team or a young disabled team. The members of the team may include a doctor specializing in the care of disabled people at home, clinical psychologists, physiotherapists, occupational therapists, speech therapists and social services social workers or care managers. The team may be able to help with your particular needs and give support to you and your family, in cooperation with your GP and the community nurse.

Palliative and hospice care

Many, but not all, hospices provide care for people with motor neurone disease. Hospices are mainly involved in the care of people with cancer, and so many people think that such care is only available to those who are soon to die. However, the aim of hospice care is to provide palliative care, which means relieving the symptoms of a disease even if the disease cannot be cured. People may be in the care of a hospice for varying periods of time, which can be for many months or years.

Palliative care can take many different forms – the care may be provided at home, in a day hospice or in a hospice unit.

With home care, teams visit and support people and their families at home. This is usually arranged with your GP and community nurse. The hospice nurse can advise on your medication and can listen to you and your family and help you all to cope with the disease and the resulting changes it brings to your lives. The nurse will visit you regularly at home and is usually part of a larger hospice team. Other members of the team may also be able to help and advise you, such as a physiotherapist, occupational therapist, social worker or counsellor and a doctor, who is often known as a consultant in palliative medicine. In some areas, the nurses are funded by the charity Macmillan Cancer Relief and are known as Macmillan nurses.

Many hospices have a day hospice or day centre that patients can attend. The centre is only open during the day, and its aim is to support people who are living at home. There is usually a nurse available to advise on difficulties you are having, and often a doctor can see you while you are at the day centre. Other members of the team are often available there too, and there are many activities to take part in, as well as the chance to have a bath or visit a hairdresser. Going to a centre allows your symptoms to be carefully assessed by the hospice team; it also gives you a chance to meet with the team and other people, and gives your family a break.

On occasion, admission to a hospice, or palliative care unit, may be helpful. Many people fear that hospices, or palliative care units, are very dismal and depressing places, with many seriously ill people and little activity. However, this is rarely the case, and the atmosphere is relaxed and welcoming. The aim is to help patients do as much as possible and to live life as fully as possible. There may be times of sadness, as in any hospital, but there is usually a very positive attitude among the members of the caring team.

Admission to a hospice may allow your various symptoms and difficulties to be eased, so that you can return home again or give you and your family a holiday during which you and they can rest and recuperate. Admission to a hospice is not necessarily a one-way ticket as many people fear.

Many hospitals now have a hospice or palliative care support team. This is a team of nurses, a doctor and, often, other professionals. The members of the team can visit patients on the main hospital wards. They can advise you, your family and the hospital doctors and nurses on your care, and help to ensure that the best preparations are made for your return home. The nurse may also be able to arrange for the home-care nurses to visit you at home or arrange your admission to a hospice if this is necessary.

The involvement of your local hospice team – at home, in hospital, in a day hospice or in a hospice itself – will help with all your problems, whether these are physical, such as pain or breathlessness, or mental, such as the fears you and your family may have about the disease and the future. Usually, a hospice team will want to meet with you in the early stages of the disease so that your symptoms and so on can be assessed and you can get to know each other. This makes it easier for you all to work together through any more difficult times. Referral to a hospice is definitely not the last step, and can be very worth-while and positive.

You may not need help from all these services at first, but as the disease progresses, it may be helpful to have further profes-sional advice. The aim in all this should always be to support you and your family, not to take over your care and reduce your independence. To achieve this, it is often very helpful if one of the professionals involved in your care becomes the key worker, someone who can coordinate the care that is offered to you and reduce the chances of something being missed or being pro-vided by several people at once. You may wish to discuss with everyone involved in your care who you would like to be your key worker and how this person would work with you and your family.

8

The role of the Motor Neurone Disease Association

Introduction

The Motor Neurone Disease Association was formed in 1979 by a group of patients and their families to share information about the disease and stimulate research into it. The Association now has over 80 branches, 7000 members and thousands of supporters, and works continuously to ensure that people affected by motor neurone disease receive the care and support they need. It also promotes and funds research into effective treatments and the search for a cure. The Association offers help in many different ways, and this chapter will show how it may be able to help you.

MND Connect – the Association's helpline

If you or any of your family or friends want to get more information about motor neurone disease, or feel the need to talk about your concerns, the number for MND Connect is 08457 626262 (all calls are charged at local rates). This helpline is open from 9 a.m. to 5 p.m. and 7 p.m. to 10.30 p.m., Monday to Friday. It is staffed by paid workers and volunteers, all specially trained. They come from a wide range of backgrounds and have often had personal experience of what living with motor neurone disease means. You will not be asked to give your name, unless you want to, and the volunteers will try to answer your questions as honestly as possible, and help you deal with concerns and issues about any aspect of motor neurone disease. The helpline can also give information in other areas such as rights to benefits and so on. As well, it can put you in touch with other professionals who may be able to help you. You can also email MND Connect via the Association's website (it is listed there under 'Contact us').

Regional care development advisers

There are regional care development advisers (RCDAs) throughout England, Wales and Northern Ireland. Their role is to ensure that you and your family receive prompt advice and support, and that you are linked up to the appropriate professional services in your area. RCDAs work very closely with Association visitors (see next section) to make sure that people affected by motor neurone disease have access to the Association's resources and the best possible care. The adviser for your area may get in touch with you directly or ensure that a local MND team, or an Association visitor, contacts you to offer support. The adviser can also provide information for your GP, community nurse and other professionals involved in your care, so that they are aware of the problems that may occur and the ways in which they can be eased or overcome. You should be asked by your local neurological centre when you are diagnosed if you would like to be put in touch with the Association locally; you can also contact it yourself via the Association's helpline or website.

The Association has developed and published its standards of care, which set out the minimum standards for the quality of care that it believes people with motor neurone disease are entitled to. Regional care development advisers have a role in educating healthcare professionals, such as doctors, nurses, physiotherapists, occupational therapists and workers in social services departments, in how to achieve these standards. They also pull together teams of these different professionals at a local level, so that all the people involved in your care are working together.

Association visitors

The Association has a network of more than 300 specially trained volunteers known as Association visitors (AVs). They are often people who have previously worked as healthcare professionals or have personal experience of the disease. The role of an AV is to befriend people with motor neurone disease and their families, by providing a listening ear, advice and support. This will vary according to what support or help you want from an AV – your AV can stay in touch by email or by phone, or meet you on a regular basis. AVs are not just there to talk about the disease; they can provide companionship and support if you are feeling lonely or isolated. AVs work closely with regional care development advisers and local branches to ensure support is available at a local level. You can contact your local AV via your local branch (see below), or through the Association's helpline.

Local branches and support groups

In many areas, there is a local branch of the Association or a support group. Each branch depends on the support of local people. Many supporters are those with the disease and their families and friends, but there are also others who want to help, including care professionals such as doctors, therapists and social workers.

There are usually regular branch meetings, which provide an opportunity to meet others and share your experiences. As motor neurone disease is not frequently encountered by many doctors and nurses, this meeting may offer you a chance to talk about the disease with those who may share your experiences and understand your concerns.

Branches also hold events to raise funds for the Association, which are then used to support people – by providing grants for holidays or respite care – or to pay for laboratory research. Branches often try to raise awareness of the disease within their local community, and fund-raising events are opportunities to publicize the work of the Association and involve local press and radio. In this way, more people become aware of the illness, and additional help may become available for those who have motor neurone disease and those who care for them. Branches may also become involved in lobbying health and social services providers for better treatment for people with the disease.

Sometimes people are unsure about going to a branch meeting, perhaps because they fear that they could see someone who is more badly affected by the disease than they are, or hear of problems that they do not have themselves – and may not even have thought of. However, most people find that the companionship and understanding that they receive when they do go overcomes such fears. Also, having a rare disease can make you feel very isolated, so it can be a very positive thing to go to a meeting and find that there are others who understand. And getting involved with helping to raise funds for care and research is one of the best ways to fight back against the disease.

Care centres

The Association has established a network of care centres to provide specialist care for people with motor neurone disease. Care centres are usually based within hospitals in various parts of the country, and aim to provide in one location all the professional care that a person with the disease needs. In this way, a number of professionals with a wide range of experience and skills in helping you live with the disease are working together, and you can see everyone you need to see during one clinic visit. In 2010, there were 18 care centres, and the aim is eventually for anyone with motor neurone disease to be less than two hours' drive from a care centre.

The centres work together, along with local carers and social services, to help to coordinate your care. They also provide centres of excellence that other neurological centres can learn from, and are often involved in clinical trials of potential future treatments.

The care service

People with motor neurone disease and those who care for them may find their lives made easier if they have access to specialist equipment, for instance a motorized riser–recliner chair, or a communication aid such as a Lightwriter. The Association supports people in getting hold of these items of equipment (which can be very expensive to buy) on a loan basis from local health and social services providers. The Association also provides equipment itself, often as a stopgap while the local service providers organize longer-term loans, or if this equipment is not available for some reason. The aim is to raise the standards of care for people with motor neurone disease by working together with health and community care providers.

The care service can also provide small grants towards the cost of care, either at home or in the form of respite care to allow carers a rest.

The national office of the Association

The national office of the Association is in Northampton (01604 250505), and it coordinates the work of all the various parts of the Association. The helpline is managed from there, and it produces a wide variety of leaflets and publications, both for people with the disease and professionals. It also runs the Association's website, and every year organizes a number of meetings and conferences for professional groups and everyone affected by motor neurone disease. Each year there is a series of spring conferences, so people affected by the disease can hear about the latest developments and thinking in care and research. Along with the AGM each September, these events also give people a chance to meet others with similar experiences and exchange ideas.

As a national charity, the Association also campaigns for better treatment for people with motor neurone disease at a national level, lobbying the government for better health policies, and representing the views of people with the disease when new legislation is being developed.

Larger-scale fund-raising activities, such as major events, corporate donations and involvement in activities like the London Marathon, are managed from the national office.

The Association also supports many research projects, both into the causes of the disease and how to treat it. These projects are carefully chosen and supervised so that the most beneficial research can take place. The financial support that the Association gives makes it the main source of funding for research into the disease in the UK.

The Association is closely linked with similar bodies in Scotland and the Irish Republic and throughout the world. Once a year it organizes an international symposium, bringing together research and care experts from across the world to share their latest developments.

The Just in Case kit

The Association developed the Just in Case kit as a result of the main concerns people voiced about how those with motor neurone disease were cared for as their condition deteriorated. Leaflets have been produced for doctors and nurses that both outline the changes that may occur as a person's condition worsens and give advice on the best ways of reducing the problems in order that the person can remain as active and comfortable as possible.

The Just in Case kit (described on page 56) is a small box that is provided by the Association to keep ready in case you suffer a choking attack or other severe difficulty with your breathing. With the box is a leaflet that gives instructions on the most suitable medication to use if this should occur. You and your family can then discuss the leaflet and the possible use of the kit with your GP and community nurse. If you all agree, the necessary medication can then be prescribed and placed in the box, so that it is readily available should a crisis occur.

The personal guide and other information

The Association produces dozens of leaflets and publications on different aspects of motor neurone disease, and you can obtain these from the national office, your local branch, or your regional care development adviser (see Further reading for a list of these publications). You can also find out information, and order leaflets, via the website (www.mndassociation.org). When reading information, it is important to remember that everyone is different and that the symptoms and difficulties described may or may not apply in your case.

The Association produces a personal guide for each person with motor neurone disease, which takes the form of a folder in which you can keep all the information you gather about the disease in one place. Many of the leaflets you can request from the Association can be clipped straight into the folder.

There is also an information pack for professionals. You should encourage your doctor, nurse or therapist to ask the Association for this professional information pack if they are unfamiliar with the disease and wish to know more about it.

Tissue donation and the DNA bank

The Association has helped to fund and coordinate research that looks into changes in the nerve cells that occur in those with the disease. This has only been possible because researchers have been able to examine the brains and spinal cords of those who have had the disease. These people and their families have given permission for this tissue to be removed after their deaths and then closely examined in a research laboratory. The necessary arrangements for moving the person who has died to the laboratory and returning them to the funeral director are all made by the laboratory (the Association can provide details of centres that can undertake this procedure). The process only takes a few hours and does not delay any other arrangements. The appearance of the person who has died is also unaffected.

In 2002 the Association established the largest ever DNA bank for motor neurone disease research. The aim is to collect DNA samples from thousands of people with and without motor neurone disease, to help carry out research into causes and treatments. Not everyone will be a suitable candidate to contribute DNA, and the Association can advise you on this.

If you and your family feel that you want to contribute to research into the disease, contact the Association for further details (see Useful addresses at the back of this book).

9

What other help is available?

Introduction

As you become less able to do the usual activities of day-to-day living, you may need extra help. This may be necessary if you are to continue to work, to live as normally as possible at home or to take a holiday. There may also be increasing financial pressures if you, and perhaps those close to you, are less able to work. This chapter aims to provide information on the practical and financial assistance that you can gain access to. Details of the various allowances from the Department of Work and Pensions (DWP) and other sources are given, but as these change periodically, do check if changes have been made before you make any claims.

At work

If you are employed when you are diagnosed as having motor neurone disease, you will need to look carefully at the future. Usually it is helpful to discuss the situation with your employer, either with your manager or someone in the personnel department. It may be possible to adjust your work or change areas of work if you are unable to continue in your present post. You may need to ask for advice from your union, works representative or occupational health adviser.

The DWP can also help you cope with changes you have to make to keep working. There are allowances to cover extra expenses you might incur travelling to work if your disability makes the journey difficult. Equipment can also be provided that will enable you to remain at work. These and other kinds of help can be discussed and claimed by you and your employer. Disablement employment advisers, who are based at Job Centres, may also be able to advise you on what you can claim or help you to look for other employment if this becomes necessary.

If you are unable to keep working, you may need to consider taking early retirement or long-term sick leave. These options should be discussed with your employer and careful consideration given to each of the choices open to you. If you take sick leave, you should be able to apply for one or more of the following benefits.

- *Statutory sick pay* This is paid by your employer. You may need to discuss this benefit and how to claim it with your employer. It is paid for a maximum of 28 weeks.
- *Employment and support allowance (ESA)* If you are unable to work as a result of illness or disability you may be able to claim ESA. In the first 13 weeks an assessment phase rate is paid while a decision is made on your capacity for work. If you are assessed as being limited in your ability to work, the main phase starts from week 14. There are payments according to your work-related activity and the support you need, based on the assessment of the severity of your disability. You may also be able to receive help with mortgage interest and housing costs.
- *Income support* If you receive statutory sick pay you may be able to receive income support as an additional benefit for the 28 weeks of the statutory sick pay. Your savings need to be below £16,000 and you need to be receiving a low income. You may also be able to receive help with mortgage interest and housing costs.
- *Incapacity benefit* This has been replaced by ESA. However, if you have claimed before October 2008 you may still be entitled to receive this benefit.

- *Housing and council tax benefit* You may be able to claim housing and council tax benefit from your local council if you receive means-tested benefit or are on a low income. This benefit will help to pay your rent and, often, council tax.

At home

Motor neurone disease will often cause disruption to life at home, and you will have increasing needs, although these will vary from person to person. There may be a need for changes to be made in the house, extra facilities or help and, also, money worries. All these changes may mean that you will need outside help to effect them, and this may come from a variety of sources – your local social services department, council, DWP and local voluntary agencies.

Housing

If the disease leads to increased disability you may need to consider making changes to the house or moving to more suitable accommodation. The council may be able to help with any such adaptations that are necessary to allow you and your family to remain in your present home and, if necessary, the council may be able to help you find somewhere better suited to your needs, including housing specially designed for disabled people. The council does have a statutory responsibility to provide appropriate housing for people with special needs, but the possibilities may be limited by financial restrictions.

Local councils have to give Disabled Facilities Grants to eligible applicants, but you may have to pay some of the costs, depending on your financial circumstances.

Your occupational therapist will be able to advise you on this whole area and help you contact your local housing department. The occupational therapist can also provide a report to support your application.

If your income has reduced, it may be possible to claim housing benefit (see page 84) from your local council. This is a means-tested allowance and is available if you are eligible for certain benefits or you are on a low income.

Other allowances

You and your family may be entitled to claim other allowances from the DWP, although you may need to show that you are eligible for some of these allowances by undergoing a means test. The following is a list of these other allowances.

- *Attendance allowance* Anyone aged 65 years or over with motor neurone disease who requires help with washing, eating, dressing or going to the toilet may be eligible for this allowance. There are two rates of payment, according to your needs. Usually there is a delay of six months before the allowance is paid. However, in cases of serious illness, you can apply under the 'special rules'. The special rules apply in cases where the illness is defined as 'terminal' and life expectancy could be less than six months. You may discuss whether or not you could claim under the special rule with your doctor, as they will need to complete a medical assessment form confirming the illness and its severity. By completing the form, the doctor is not necessarily confirming that you will be *likely* to die within the next six months, but only that this is possible. If you apply under the special rules, there is *no* delay in the payments being made and you will receive the first one within a few weeks. The attendance allowance is not means tested, or taxed, and does not affect any claims for other allowances, such as income support and housing benefit.

- *Pension credit* If you have reached the minimum qualifying age, the DWP may assess whether you qualify for this means-tested benefit. It has two parts:
  - *The guarantee credit*, which replaced income support (the age at which you can claim is gradually being increased from 60 to 65 years between 2010 and 2020), and
  - *The savings credit* for people aged 65 and over, which is intended to provide extra money for people with modest savings.

Pension credit can also meet mortgage payments and other housing costs.

- *Disability living allowance* If you are under 65 years old, you may apply for disability living allowance instead of attendance allowance. The claim is processed in the same way, but you may receive an extra payment if you require help with getting about. For this payment, you need to fill in an additional form, giving details of your disability and mobility needs. A medical assessment may be necessary. The allowance is similar to the attendance allowance, but it is payable when you have needed help for only three months. It may also be claimed under the special rules (see 'Attendance allowance' above). It is not means tested, or taxed, and does not affect other benefits.
- *Carer's allowance* This allowance is paid to the carers of someone who is receiving attendance allowance or disability living allowance. Your carer must be aged 16 years or over and would need to show that he or she is spending over 35 hours a week looking after you. It is possible to claim this allowance and continue working, if your earnings are less than £100 a week. This allowance *is* taxed and taken into account when other benefits, such as income support and housing benefit, are calculated. The person receiving the allowance is credited with Class 1 National Insurance contributions, as if in paid employment.

- *Carer's credit* If you do not qualify for the carer's allowance or means-tested benefit, you may be eligible for this, which helps to protect your right to a state pension. If you are caring for someone who receives disability living allowance or attendance allowance, you may have to apply every year to say that you wish to receive this protection.
- *Child tax credit* This is a means-tested or income-related payment for people who are responsible for a child, whether in or out of work. The claim is for a child up to 16 years old or, in some circumstances, a child aged 16 to 19 years old who is in full-time, non-advanced education.
- *Working tax credit* This is a means-tested or income-related payment for those in low-paid work. You need to work a minimum of 16 hours per week to claim if you have children, or over 30 hours per week if you are over 25 and do not have children. Payments can also be made towards certain child-care costs.

Both child tax credit and working tax credit are tax-free and administered by the Inland Revenue.

The Social Fund

If you are receiving income support, income-based jobseekers' allowance, income-related employment and support allowance or pension credit, this fund is available to help you if you find it difficult to pay for your expenses out of your regular income. Payments made to you do not depend on your National Insurance contributions. There are various such payments that may be claimed.

- *Community care grant* This may be claimed to help you stay at home or to help relieve pressure on your family. A grant may be made for furniture, removal costs, minor house repairs or certain travel costs.

- *Budgeting and crisis loans* A budgeting loan is an interest-free loan that may be given to allow you to buy a necessity, such as a new cooker or bed. A crisis loan may be claimed if you need something quickly. The loans have to be repaid, but the *rate* of repayment is calculated by taking into account your income and expenses.

Other help

- *Prescription exemption* If you are over 60 years old, you will not have to pay for your prescriptions. If you are under 60 years old, you will have to pay prescription costs, unless you claim exemption because you have a low income and receive income support or have a 'continuing physical disability which prevents you from leaving home except with the help of another person'. If eligible, you need to fill in the form (available from your doctor or a pharmacist, a post office, a social security officer or Family Health Services Authority office). If you are *not* eligible for exemption from prescription charges, you may benefit from buying a prepayment certificate. This allows you to obtain as many prescriptions as necessary during the period covered by the certificate without having to make any further payment.
- *Dental charges* If you have a low income, you may be able to receive free NHS dental treatment or reduced charges. Anyone receiving income support will automatically receive free dental treatment.
- *Fares to hospital* You may be eligible for help with fares to hospital for regular appointments or treatment if you have a low income and, on occasion, a person travelling with you may also be able to claim their fares. Visitors coming to see you in hospital may also claim for their expenses if they are receiving a means-tested benefit. A claim is made for a community care grant from the Social Fund.

Many of these allowances and benefits may seem confusing and complicated. If you find that it is difficult to make the claims, contact your local social security office (the address will be in the telephone book under Department of Work and Pensions) or your care manager or social worker from social services for advice. There are also free telephone helplines (Benefit Enquiry Line 0800 882200). Leaflets on these subjects are often available at post offices. You may also find that your local Citizens' Advice Bureau or legal centre may be able to help you.

Your care manager or social worker from the local social services department will also be able to advise you on the provision of extra help at home, and can also be a source of good advice if you and your family are considering your going into a residential home or nursing home, for either a period of respite care or for longer-term care (see pages 60–1).

Getting around

If you are 65 years old or under, you may be able to claim the mobility component of disability living allowance (see page 84). You will need to complete the form giving details of your needs. If you are in doubt as to whether or not you are eligible, ask at the DWP, ask your care manager or ring the Benefit Enquiry Line.

If you receive the higher rate of this mobility component, you may use this allowance to hire a car through Motability, a non-profitmaking organization. You can choose a car to buy or to hire from a wide range of models. Your mobility component is then paid to Motability and you may have to make an additional payment, according to the car that you have chosen. You and one other person may drive the car and, if you are unable to drive, you may nominate two drivers. The Motability scheme can also be used to buy a powered wheelchair that suits your needs on hire purchase. To contact them, write to Motability, Motability Operations, City Gate House, 22 Southwark Bridge Road, London SE1 9HB (telephone: 0845 456 4566; website: www.motability.co.uk).

You may also be able to apply for other help if you are disabled, such as the following.

- *Blue Badge* The local authority may be able to issue you with a Blue Badge, which allows you to park in designated parking spaces for the disabled, to park for longer periods and free of charge at parking meters and pay and display on-street parking, and to park for up to three hours on single or double lines, except where there is a ban on loading and unloading or where the car would cause an obstruction. You can apply to your local social services department for the badge if you are receiving disability living allowance or attendance allowance with the mobility component, or your doctor will confirm that you have a 'permanent and substantial disability which means that you are unable to work or have considerable difficulty in walking'.
- *Vehicle excise duty* You may not have to pay this duty if you are receiving disability living allowance and it includes the mobility component.
- *Car purchase or adaptation* If you purchase a car through the Motability scheme or otherwise purchase a car and are a wheelchair user, you will not have to pay car tax or VAT. If you are registered disabled, you do not have to pay VAT on adaptations made to your car either.
- *Public transport* Many bus companies and National Rail offer reduced fares for disabled people. Passengers in wheelchairs pay less on trains, and there is a disabled persons railcard that allows you to travel for reduced fares.
- *ServiceCall* A ServiceCall transmitter is one that can be used

from your car to attract the attention of staff in shops, banks or petrol stations. The transmitter sends out a signal that is picked up by a receiver in the shop. A member of staff will then come to assist you. When you apply to have a transmitter, you can inform ServiceCall of the local shops, banks, petrol stations or other places that you visit regularly, and ServiceCall will arrange for a receiver to be fitted at these places. To contact them, write to ServiceCall, Milford Lane, Bakewell, Derbyshire DE45 1EX, or telephone them on 01629 814488 (Freephone: 0800 458 3008, email: info@service-call. net; website: www.service-call.net).

Holidays

Finding suitable holiday accommodation may be difficult for you and your family as you become less mobile. Advice on holidays is available from the following organizations.

- *The Royal Association for Disability Rights* The Association publishes two guides for disabled people – 'Holidays in the British Isles' and 'Holidays and Travel Abroad'. It can be contacted by writing to 12 City Forum, 250 City Road, London EC1V 8AF, phoning 020 7250 3222, or visiting their website: www. radar.org.uk.
- *The Automobile Association* The AA produces the 'AA Disabled Travellers' Guide', which is free to members.
- *Travel agents* Many travel agents will be able to advise you as to the accessibility of holiday accommodation and on holidays that will not make life difficult for you. However, it is very important to ensure that the agent is aware of *all* your needs and that they check that these will be met before the booking is made.
- *Your local social services department* You may be able to get good advice from this source – and find out if it is possible for you to get a grant towards your holiday costs. Your local

branch of the Motor Neurone Disease Association may also be able to give you such a grant.

- *Holiday insurance* Most holiday insurance policies will not cover you when you have a serious illness such as motor neurone disease. You will need to check with the insurance company and, if you are *not* covered, contact the Motor Neurone Disease Association for details of companies that will provide cover. If you are travelling abroad it is essential for you to have adequate medical insurance, as the costs of seeing a doctor or admission to hospital could be substantial.

The Citizens' Advice Bureau

The Citizens' Advice Bureau is able to offer independent and reliable advice on a wide range of matters, including local facilities, services and finance. The staff are trained in providing information for you and can call on specialized advice if necessary. You will find details of your local Citizens' Advice Bureau in the telephone book, under Citizens' Advice Bureau.

Patient Advice and Liaison Services

If you have experienced difficulties with the care you have received from the medical and nursing services, you may contact the Patient Advice and Liaison Services (PALS). PALS are available in every NHS Trust and can provide:

- confidential advice and support to patients, families and carers
- information on the NHS and health-related matters
- confidential assistance in resolving problems and concerns quickly.

PALS are independent of NHS Trusts and can liaise with staff and managers to resolve problems. They can be contacted by telephoning the hospital, GP surgery or health centre, or by telephoning NHS Direct (0845 46 47).

In all NHS Trusts there are also Patient and Public Involvement Forums, which are involved in:

- monitoring and reviewing services
- seeking the views of patients
- promoting the involvement of the public in healthcare developments.

They can be contacted by telephoning the NHS Trust concerned.

Useful addresses

There are many other voluntary groups that can provide advice and help to you and your family. There are sometimes large, national organizations, or there may be local groups that you can join. Some groups may offer very specialized advice and may not be able to provide help to everyone with motor neurone disease. I have tried to include as many groups as possible that may be of help.

AbilityNet
AbilityNet Thames Valley
c/o Microsoft Ltd
Microsoft Campus
Thames Valley Park
Reading RG6 1WG
Tel.: 01926 312847
Freephone: 0800 269545
Website: www.abilitynet.org.uk
A national charity offering advice and help on the use of computers for disabled people.

Age UK
Adviceline: 0800 169 6565
Website: www.ageuk.org.uk
Age UK aims to improve later life for everyone through information and support.

Age UK England
Astral House
1268 London Road
London SW16 4ER
Tel.: 020 8765 7200

Age UK Northern Ireland
3 Lower Crescent
Belfast BT7 1NR
Tel.: 028 9024 5729

Age UK Scotland
Causewayside House
160 Causewayside
Edinburgh EH9 1PR
Tel.: 0845 125 9732

Age UK Wales
Tŷ John Pathy
13–14 Neptune Court
Vanguard Way
Cardiff CF24 5PJ
Tel.: 029 2043 1555

British Red Cross
44 Moorfields
London EC2Y 9AL
Tel.: 0844 871 1111
Website: www.redcross.org.uk
The Red Cross can provide equipment, such as wheelchairs and commodes, via their medical equipment service. There are also schemes that provide trained and supervised helpers who are able to care for you and allow your carers a rest. There is also a transport and escort service, providing an ambulance and car service, and helpers to travel with you if necessary.

Carers UK
20 Great Dover Street
London SE1 4LX
Tel.: 020 7378 4999
Advice line: 0808 808 7777 (10 a.m. to 12 p.m. and 2 to 4 p.m., Wednesdays and Thursdays)
Website: www.carersuk.org
This association aims to support anyone caring for someone who is ill or disabled by encouraging carers to recognize their own needs, providing information and advice, and bringing the needs of carers to the attention of government and policy makers. It produces leaflets and runs carers' support groups.

Crossroads Care
10 Regent Place
Rugby
Warwickshire CV21 2PN
Tel.: 0845 450 0350
Website: www.crossroads.org.uk
Crossroads Care provides support and help in the home for carers.

Cruse Bereavement Care
PO Box 800
Richmond
Surrey TW9 2RG
Tel.: 020 8939 9530
Daytime helpline: 0844 477 9400 (9.30 a.m. to 5 p.m., Monday to Friday)
Young person's helpline (Freephone): 0808 808 1677
Website: www.crusebereavementcare.org.uk
Cruse Bereavement Care offers help to all bereaved people by providing
counselling, advice and information on practical matters and
opportunities to meet with others.

DIAL UK
St Catherine's
Tickhill Road
Doncaster
South Yorkshire DN4 8QN
Tel.: 01302 310123
website: www.dialuk.info
The DIAL network consists of over 120 local disability information and
advice services. Trained advice workers can offer advice on a range of
topics related to disability.

Disability Alliance
Universal House
88–94 Wentworth Street
London E1 7SA
Tel.: 020 7247 8776
Website: www.disabilityalliance.org
Disability Alliance researches the needs of the disabled and campaigns
both for improvements in the living standards of disabled people and for
a greater understanding of their needs. Its *Disability Rights Handbook* is a
guide to all available state benefits.

Disabled Living Foundation
380–384 Harrow Road
London W9 2HU
Tel.: 020 7289 6111
Helpline: 0845 130 9177 (10 a.m. to 4 p.m., Monday to Friday)
Website: www.dlf.org.uk
Provides information on the various aids and appliances available for
disabled people. At the Foundation professional help and advice is
available and aids can be seen and tried. An appointment is necessary.

Irish MND Association
Coleraine House
Coleraine Street
Dublin 7
Freephone: 1800 403 403
Website: www.imnda.ie

Jewish Care
Merit House
508 Edgware Road
London NW9 5AB
Tel.: 020 8922 2000
Helpline: 020 8922 2222
Website: www.jewishcare.org
Jewish Care provides help for people within the Jewish community,
offering residential, respite and day care and outreach services for younger
disabled people. There are home-care visitors, social workers
and volunteer visitors throughout the country, as well as carer support
groups.

Leonard Cheshire Disability
66 South Lambeth Road
London SW8 1RL
Tel.: 020 3242 0200
Website: www.lcdisability.org
Supports disabled people in the UK and across the world, campaigns for
change and provides innovative services that give disabled people the
opportunity to live life their way. Services include care homes, supported
living, domiciliary support, day services, resource centres, rehabilitation,
respite care, personal care and training and assistance for those looking
for work.

Livability
50 Scrutton Street
London EC2A 4XQ
Tel.: 020 7452 2000
Website: www.livability.org.uk
Aims to help disabled people by providing wheelchair-accessible
accommodation and residential homes, help with care at home, a hotel
and travel service and (for some) employment.

Mobilise
Ashwellthorpe
Norwich NR16 1EX
Tel.: 01508 489449
Website: www.mobilise.info
Mobilise is a UK charity that promotes mobility for all disabled people. It provides an information and support service for members; its information officers can offer help and advice on a range of issues, including parking, vehicle adaptations, the Blue Badge scheme, public transport, scooters and wheelchairs, exemption from vehicle excise duty and access issues. It also publishes a monthly magazine and campaigns nationally on many issues that affect disabled people, including congestion charging, pedestrianization, abuse of disabled bays and accessibility of goods and services.

MND Scotland
76 Firhill Road
Glasgow G20 7BA
Tel.: 0141 945 1077
Website: www.mndscotland.org.uk

Motor Neurone Disease Association
PO Box 246
Northampton NN1 2PR
Tel.: 01604 250505
MND Connect (helpline): 08457 626262
Website: www.mndassociation.org

RADAR: The Disability Network
12 City Forum
250 City Road
London EC1V 8AF
Tel.: 020 7250 3222
Website: www.radar.org.uk
RADAR is a pressure group working to improve the rights and needs of disabled people. It monitors current and proposed legislation and produces information and advice on all issues related to disability.

Sex and Disability Helpline
Dr Tuppy Owens
BCM Box Lovely
London WC1N 3XX
Tel.: 070 7499 3527 (11 a.m. to 7 p.m., Monday to Friday)
Website: www.outsiders.org.uk
The Sex and Disability Helpline is available for advice, and leaflets are available on various aspects of sexuality and disability.

Tourism for All
c/o Vitalise
Shap Road Industrial Estate
Shap Road
Kendal
Cumbria LA9 6NZ
Tel.: 0845 124 9971
Website: www.tourismforall.org.uk
Produces information on holiday accommodation for disabled people, including accessible hotels, farmhouses, guest houses and self-catering accommodation, transport, organized holidays and holidays where care is provided.

Other useful websites

The following websites provide information for people with MND, their families and professional carers.

www.alsa.org
The US amyotrophic lateral sclerosis (ALS) association, with a great deal of information.

www.alsmndalliance.org
The international alliance of MND/ALS associations. Includes a directory of MND/ALS societies worldwide.

www.wfnals.org
The World Federation of Neurology Research Group on MND and ALS. An excellent site with regularly updated clinico-scientific news on MND/ALS and a worldwide list of MND/ALS specialists and centres.

Further reading

The Motor Neurone Disease Association produces many leaflets and also provides information:

The Personal Guide to MND
An A4 binder including a range of practical advice and information. There are optional sections that can be added:

- Carers
- Children and young people
- Everyday activities
- More about MND – types, tests and treatments
- Symptoms
- Movement and mobility
- Speech and communication
- Eating and drinking
- End-of-life decisions
- Symptoms.

There are also information sheets:

- Clothing ideas
- Kennedy's disease
- Holiday and travel information
- Motoring and MND
- Motor insurance
- MND statistics
- Riluzole – questions and answers
- Equipment provision by the Motor Neurone Disease Association
- PEG feeding: making the decision
- Oral hygiene
- Complementary therapies

- Understanding how MND might affect your breathing
- Ventilation in MND.

MND Association leaflets and booklets:

- Troubleshooting and NIV
- Air travel and NIV
- Primary lateral sclerosis
- NMD Care Centre programme
- Progressive muscular atrophy
- Advance decision to refuse treatment explained
- Advance decision to refuse treatment – full pack
- Sex and relationships
- Physiotherapy for people with MND
- Cognitive impairment in MND
- So what is MND anyway? A guide for young people
- When someone close has MND: a workbook for children aged 4–10.

Other leaflets, etc. include:

- Recipe collection: easy-to-swallow meals
- Notepad for people with speech difficulties, each page headed with:
  'I can understand you but have difficulty speaking, please read on'
- Speech card for people with speech difficulties (credit card size): *'I have a physical problem which affects my speech, but I can hear and understand you. Your help and patience would be appreciated. Thank you'.*

These leaflets are updated regularly and further details and ordering is from the MND Association.

Books

Albom, M., *Tuesdays with Morrie*, Doubleday, 1997
Mitsumoto, M. D. and Munsat, T. L., *Amyotrophic Lateral Sclerosis: A guide for patients and families*, Demos, 2001, 2nd edition

Neilson, S. and Clifford Rose, F. *Motor Neurone Disease: The 'at your fingertips' guide*, Class Publishing, 2003

Pegg, S., *Just Some Stories for Eleanor*, Doubleday, 1991

For professional workers

Belsh, J. and Schiffman, P., *Amyotrophic Lateral Sclerosis: Diagnosis and management for the clinician*, Futura, 1996

Brown, R. H., Meininger, V. and Swash, M., *Amyotrophic Lateral Sclerosis*, Martin Dunitz, 2000

Kuncl, R. W. (ed.), *Motor Neuron Disease*, W. B. Saunders, 2002

Leigh, P. and Swash, M.(eds), *Motor Neuron Disease: Biology and management*, Springer-Verlag, 1995

Mitsumoto, H. and Norris, F. H., *Amyotrophic Lateral Sclerosis: A comprehensive guide to management*, Demos, 1994

MND Resource File: A patient and carer centred approach for health and social care professionals, MND Association, 2000

Motor Neurone Disease: A problem solving approach for general practitioners and the primary health care team, MND Association, 1996

Oliver, D., Borasio, G. D. and Walsh, D. (eds), *Palliative Care in Amyotrophic Lateral Sclerosis: From diagnosis to bereavement*, second edition, Oxford University Press, 2000

Oliver, D., *Motor Neurone Disease*, Royal College of General Practitioners, 1994, 2nd edition

Resources for ALS Healthcare Providers, ALS Society of Canada, 1994

Voltz, R., Borasio, G. D., Bernat, J., Maddocks, I., Oliver, D. and Portenoy, R. K. (eds), *Palliative Care in Neurology*, Oxford University Press, 2004

Index

advance care planning 56–8
allowances 44, 85–8
anxiety 33–4

bed sores 33
blood test 11
bowels 32
brain scan 13
breathing 23–4, 47–50; exercises
  24; non-invasive ventilation
  24, 48–9, 52

care needs 43–5, 59–61, 62–74;
  hospital care 62–3; *see also*
  advance care planning
children 37–9, 66; *When Someone
  Close Has MND* workbook 38
choking 55–6; *see also* Just in
  Case kit
cognitive change 53
communication 26–9; equipment
  28, 29, 78; telephone 28; *see
  also* speech and language
  therapy
confusion 52–3
counselling 14, 34, 65–6
crying 33

depression 33–4
dietitian 24, 26, 70; *see also*
  swallowing
dribbling *see* swallowing
driving 89–91
dying 54–5

electromyography (EMG) 12

family 15, 16–17, 35–45, 56, 66
finances 42–3, 82–4; *see also*
  allowances

general practitioner (GP) 10–17,
  64–5
genetics 7, 41–2; *see also* motor
  neurone disease: familial MND

holidays 82, 91–2
hospice and palliative care 60,
  71–3; *see also* care needs
housing 67–8, 84–5; *see also*
  allowances

incontinence 54

Just in Case kit 56, 79–80

key worker 15, 73

lumbar puncture 12

magnetic resonance imaging
  (MRI) scan 12
medication 22–3, 24, 25, 31, 32,
  34, 52, 58–9; Just in Case kit
  56, 79–80; morphine 31, 47–8;
  syringe driver 59
Mental Capacity Act 56–7; *see
  also* advance care planning
motor neurone disease (MND):
  amyotrophic lateral sclerosis 3,
  20, 100; causes 7–9; drug trials
  18–21; early stages 5–6; familial
  MND 41; fasciculation 3, 6;

progressive bulbar palsy 3–4;
progressive muscular atrophy
4; research 18, 78, 79, 81; *see
also* Motor Neurone Disease
Association
Motor Neurone Disease
Association 14, 17, 44, 64,
74–82; Association visitors
76; care centres 77–8; funding
research 81; local branches
44–5; national office 78–9,
99; personal guide folder 80;
regional care development
advisers 14, 44, 75–6; *When
Someone Close Has MND*
(children's workbook) 38
muscle biopsy 13

neurologist 10, 11, 14, 62
nurse: community nurse 43, 65;
hospital nurse 63–4

occupational therapy 14–15, 30,
47, 66, 67–8, 75

pain 22–3; *see also* medication:
morphine
percutaneous endoscopic
gastrostomy (PEG) (tube
feeding) 26, 50–1
percutaneous radiological

gastrostomy (PRG) (tube
feeding) 51–2
physical disability team 70
physiotherapy 14, 23, 24, 29,
30, 31, 46–7, 68–9, 75; *see also*
rehabilitation consultant
prescriptions 88

radiologically inserted
gastrostomy (RIG) *see*
percutaneous radiological
gastrostomy (PRG)
rehabilitation consultant 14, 63
research *see* motor neurone
disease: drug trials, research

sex 39–41
sleeping 31–2, 48
social worker 14, 34, 43, 44,
65–6, 89
speech and language therapy 15,
24, 26, 27, 69–70
stiffness 22–3, 31
swallowing 24–6, 50–2

tissue donation 81

walking 29–30
weakness 29–30, 46–7
wheelchair 30, 47
work 82–3; *see also* allowances